HEALTHY

HEALTH

About the Authors

Maryon Stewart studied preventative dentistry and nutrition at the Royal Dental Hospital in London and worked as a counsellor with nutritional doctors in England for four years. At the beginning of 1984 she set up the PMT Advisory Service which has subsequently helped thousands of women world-wide. In 1987 she launched the Women's Nutritional Advisory Service which now provides broader help to women of all ages.

Maryon Stewart is the author of the best-selling books *Beat PMS Through Diet*, now in its third edition, *Beat Sugar Craving*, and *Beat the Menopause Without HRT*. She is the co-author of *The Vitality Diet*, *Beat IBS Through Diet* and *The PMT Cookbook*. She has had her own weekly radio programme on health and nutrition, she has co-written several medical papers, and has written articles for many glossy magazines and for the *Daily Mirror*. She has also appeared on several popular TV magazine shows, has contributed regularly to 'Capital Woman', has done a series of programmes for Yorkshire TV's 'Help Yourself' programmes and has helped Anglia TV with their 'Bodyworks' series. Maryon has written her own regular page in the magazine *House and Garden* and she now writes regularly for *Health and Fitness* magazine. She is on the Panel of Advisors for *First Steps* magazine and frequently lectures to both the lay public and medical profession. She is married to Dr Alan Stewart and they live in Lewes, Sussex, with their four children.

Dr Alan Stewart qualified as a doctor at Guy's Hospital, London, in 1976 and spent five years specialising in hospital medicine. He is a member of the Royal College of Physicians.

He worked at the Royal London Homeopathic Hospital and qualified as a Member of the Faculty of Homoeopathy. Since then he has specialised in nutritional medicine, and was a founding member of the British Society for Nutritional Medicine. He is also a medical advisor to the Women's Nutritional Advisory Service, and is actively involved in educating other doctors on the subject of nutrition. Dr Stewart co-wrote the best-selling books *Nutritional Medicine, Beat IBS Through Diet* and *The Vitality Diet*, he wrote *Tired All The Time*, and has contributed to other books, including *Beat PMS Through Diet, Beat Sugar Craving, Inside Science, The Migraine Revolution, The Sinclair Diet System*, and the academic book *Post Viral Fatigue Syndrome*. He has written several medical papers and regularly gives lectures to doctors and health visitors. He has also written articles in both the medical and popular press on various aspects of health, and now writes the doctor page for *Healthy Eating* magazine. He has contributed to many radio programmes and appeared on many TV magazine shows and documentaries.

HEALTHY PARENTS, HEALTHY BABY

Maryon Stewart

with contributions from
Dr Alan Stewart

Foreword by Rosie Barnes
Director of WellBeing

HEADLINE

To Phoebe, Chesney, Hester, Simeon, Emile
and Chessca, the parents of tomorrow.

'If we care about our health, and the health of the next generation, we should remember that good food is fundamental to good health.'
Caroline Walker

CONTENTS

PART THREE Healthy Baby

APPENDICES

ACKNOWLEDGEMENTS

Before even beginning to thank the people that assisted me with this book, I must mention some of the pioneers whose research I have found utterly inspiring. Margaret and Arthur Wynn, who have dedicated at least the last twenty years to demonstrating the vital need for adequate pre-conception care, have my unreserved respect. May they live to be 120 in good health. Stephen Wynn and Wendy Doyle have continued to prove the association between maternal diet and birth dimensions. Professor David Barker, together with colleagues at Southampton University, have demonstrated to the scientific world that nutrition of both the unborn and the new-born baby has significant effect on the health of the adult. Doctors Penny and Andrew Stanway have written brilliant books, and their campaigning efforts have resulted in vastly increased numbers of healthy babies. The National Childbirth Trust disseminate vital research and support women in the act of reproducing and breast-feeding their children. Nim Barnes of Foresight, the charity for preconceptual care, is acknowledged for her dedication in helping prospective parents to have healthier babies. My admiration goes to Rosie Barnes and her team at WellBeing, whose efforts fund vital medical research in hospitals and universities all over the country into better health for women and their babies. Dr Stephen Davies, by providing the facilities of his laboratory, Biolab, has made it possible for us to detect nutritional deficiencies and correct them. And, finally Caroline Walker, food writer and campaigner, who sadly died long before her time. She dedicated her life to the promotion of public health by means of good food; she influenced the course of my life greatly, and I feel privileged to have known her.

I am very grateful to Irene Duncan at *First Steps* magazine for providing the platform for our survey, and to Valerie Duncan for all her practical help and support. And grateful thanks are due to Sanatogen and Kimberly-Clark for providing the funds to enable us to conduct the survey.

Next I must thank my dedicated team at the Women's Nutritional Advisory Service for their help with this book, in particular Cheryl Griffiths who helps me to see the light at the end of the tunnel, and Ingrid Wood for stepping in to help with the data entry the survey which involved working long hours in a short space of time.

Thanks are also due to Lavinia Trevor, my agent, for her wisdom and continued support, to Sue Fleming for her inspiring editing, and to Roger Houghton at Headline for his professionalism and constant sense of humour.

My mother Rosa deserves a medal for coping with our four children whilst I was absent writing, especially as our youngest son was going through his Batman phase at the time! And my thanks are due to the children them-selves, who were unbelievably accommodating whilst they patiently waited for me to complete this book so that we could go on our much planned holiday.

Last but by no means least is untold gratitude to my husband Dr Alan Stewart, who is undoubtedly my best friend. He has contributed to this book, looked after me whilst I was writing, cooked me excellent meals, given me regular back rubs and words of encouragement, and as usual keeps me 'on the straight and narrow'.

PLEASE NOTE

As I have had two boys and two girls myself I always find books that only refer to an unborn baby as 'he' or 'she' irritating. After deliberating about how to get around this problem. I decided that it would be simpler if I referred to the prospective baby as 'she' in some chapters and 'he' in others. I hope you find this acceptable.

Foreword by Rosie Barnes

Director of WellBeing

I first met Maryon Stewart and her husband Alan in the House of Common's Tea Room, soon after I became a Member of Parliament in 1987. They had recently launched the Women's Nutritional Advisory Service, and had asked to come and see me to persuade me of the importance of diet and nutrition in relation to health problems, and to women's health in particular. They were preaching to the converted. I had realised for some time that diet and health were inextricably linked, not just in the obvious way in that a poor diet is likely to lead to poor health, but also in a much more subtle way. I had recognised in myself, in my own family and in discussion with friends that we would improve and to some extent control our own well-being by what we ate.

This had struck me forcibly after my first baby was born, in 1973, when I suffered from alopaecia, which is characterised by large, shiny bald patches. I was referred for conventional medical treatment and found myself even more depressed when I was given a greasy cream to rub into the scalp. Insult was rather added to injury when, besides the bald patches, I had greasy, lank locks instead of my former crowning glory. And all to no avail. The alopaecia did not get better and may in fact have got slightly worse. I was somewhat cynical when given an article by a kindly vegetarian friend from a health magazine suggesting treatment for alopaecia which I remember included no animal fats, lots of leeks and large doses of brewer's yeast! In spite of being dubious about its likely success I was quite prepared to give it a try, and to my surprise, and delight, soft down started to appear on the shiny bald skin.

It could of course have been coincidence, but ever since then I have been prepared to try and help myself and indeed my family to overcome health problems and to maximise our well-being by self-help methods, including diet, before resorting to the doctor. Indeed when old wives' tales handed down over generations, with simple remedies for common complaints such as cranberry juice for cystitis, are subjected to scientific research, the results, as in this example, are often positive. Cranberry juice was shown to strip the bladder of the build up of the bacteria in which cystitis thrives.

So back in 1987 when Maryon Stewart explained the principles of her Nutritional Advisory Service to me, I was very happy to endorse and support it.

Since then our lives have converged again. As director of WellBeing, the Health Research Charity for Women and Babies, I am involved in raising funds for vital medical research. As the research arm of the Royal College of Obstetricians and Gynaecologists, we are particularly interested in nutrition in pregnancy. We have funded much invaluable research in this area and in the light of results to date, we hope to be in a position to be able to significantly expand our programme of nutritional research.

The importance of this work can not be overemphasised. I recently wrote an article "You Are What Your Mother Ate". In view of the results of recent research, I should soon be able to write a sequel, "You Are What Your Grandmother Ate".

We are constantly learning more about the subtle and complex ways we are affected by what we do and do not eat throughout our lives. As women, our menstrual cycle and problems associated with it such as pre-menstrual tension are clearly influenced by our diet. It is not only pregnant women who get food cravings. Women approaching their monthly period often get desperate for sweet, starchy food and chocolate in particular. We learn that evening primrose oil such as Efamol can help to alleviate the breast pain often experienced at this time. So it is hardly surprising to discover that at the time of conception, what we do and don't consume can have significant consequences. Fertilisation and the early development of a baby are controlled by delicately balanced chemical processes. Additional chemicals entering the baby, including medication can upset this development. Similarly the lack of nutrients can have serious long term effects.

We all know that well-nourished, healthy mums are likely to produce bonnier babies than under-nourished women in poor health. It is common sense really. However what we did not know until recently was just how important nutrition is, not just during pregnancy, but before conception even occurs, and not just to help produce a healthy baby, but to ensure good health in adult life. We now know that the foundation of problems such as heart disease, diabetes and strokes are often laid down in pregnancy. We think that the reason for this is that in times of food shortage or even starvation, the baby's developing brain is given priority over other parts of the body such as the heart or the liver, so these organs develop poorly. We also know that a baby's health can be affected by the lack of vital nutrients at the time of conception. So it is not just the growing baby that needs good food, but even tiny embryos. Folic acid is known to be particularly important in this respect, helping to prevent neural tube defects such as spina bifida.

So without losing sight of the fact that pregnancy should be a happy and relaxed time, it is vitally important to consider what you eat when thinking about having a baby. Even if you have never given much thought to what you ate before, now is the time to eat a healthy, well-balanced diet in order to give yourself and your baby the best possible start.

In doing what is best for you and your baby, it is easy to get obsessional. It is also easy to make yourself miserable and anxious if you think you have eaten the wrong things or not eaten the right things. There is no place for guilt in all of this. It is quite easy to eat a healthy and well-balanced diet and to enjoy it and what is more, to have fun as well. If you find yourself pregnant but have never given a moment's thought to folic acid – and quite possibly you have never even heard of it – don't panic. You can start to take a folic acid supplement straight away, but as most Kellogg's cereals, quite a lot of brown breads as well as potatoes and green vegetables, especially broccoli, are rich in folic acid, the likelihood is that you have had a reasonable amount without ever knowing it.

Once you know you are pregnant, you will want to do what is best for both of you. Maryon Stewart's book is easy to read and full of answers. By helping you to help not only yourself, not only your unborn baby, but also the adult your baby will become, and quite probably your grandchildren as well, the well-being of several generations will be enhanced by your understanding of the importance of good food.

London
June 1995

INTRODUCTION

Pregnancy is not just about sex, round tummies, food cravings and labour pains. When we decide to have a family, we are producing part of the next generation, which is surely one of the most important jobs in the world. Mother Nature, in her great wisdom, creates the environment in which the baby can grow, and provides us with breast-milk, the perfect food to nourish the baby during its first months. However, research now shows that she needs a helping hand, as the nutritional shape that both parents are in – *at least four months prior to conception* – will determine not only the health and well-being of the new-born baby, but also its chances of health in adult life.

You no doubt know that it takes both an ovum, an egg from an ovary, and a sperm to make a baby. But did you know that both eggs and sperm may be adversely affected by inadequate diet, and by social substances like tobacco and alcohol, drugs and chemicals, environmental factors and certain viruses? The egg is at its most vulnerable for about 100 days leading up to ovulation, the time when it is released. Particularly critical times occur when the egg is undergoing changes, about three days before ovulation and on the day of fertilisation itself. Sperms are also particularly vulnerable for approximately 116 days before they mature.

As prospective parents our general health, dietary habits

1

and fitness level all play a major part in influencing the health outcome of our unborn children. Human beings are products of forty-six cycles of cell division, forty-two of which occur before birth. So eating well and being on your best behaviour both before and during pregnancy is essential to ensure that you make a healthy baby – and then adult. As fully responsible prospective parents you will both need to plan in advance, and make the changes to your diet and lifestyle at least four months before conception.

But it doesn't end there. We now know that the type of diet our babies are fed during the first year of life will also play a major part in determining their long-term health prospects. You will need to fully appreciate the advantages of breast-feeding, and then learn what to feed your baby during the weaning process. For example, if your baby becomes iron deficient she may develop anaemia and have growth and learning disorders. If on the other hand you feed your baby the wrong type of food too soon, she could develop allergies in later life, or coeliac disease.

By making sure that our eggs and sperm are in tip-top shape *before* pregnancy, that we eat well *during* pregnancy, and that we provide our new babies with the best possible diet during that vital first year of life, we will be minimising their future risk of heart disease, stroke, diabetes, high blood pressure and cholesterol levels, as well as favourably influencing their intelligence and physical abilities!

These new research findings place a great deal of responsibility on health-care professionals to convey the correct message, but the bottom line is that it is down to us as individuals to gather the data and act on it. If we knew in advance that the quality of our future children's health depended upon the shape that we ourselves are in prior to pregnancy, and certainly throughout pregnancy, there would undoubtedly be a greater quest for information. In fact many of us would be knocking doors down in order to get educated.

2

Pregnancy and motherhood often come as a complete shock to new mothers, despite the fact that women have been experiencing pregnancy, childbirth and the rearing of children since time began. There is no job description available for you to browse through before taking the plunge, so the purpose of this book is to provide you with all the information you are likely to need in order to make a healthy baby, and to preserve your sanity as you go through each vital stage.

The book is in three parts. The first is a round-up of all the latest information on pre-conception, with step-by-step advice and a complete programme for both you and your partner to follow. The second part deals with pregnancy, giving details about the new research, with a detailed programme and dietary regime for you to follow. The third part deals with the feeding options for a new baby, and how to safely wean your baby during the crucial stages of development. There are some simple sample menus for you to experiment with also. At the end of the book there are appendices which contain many useful addresses and a list of highly recommended further reading.

By following the advice in this book, you will not only be helping your baby and the next generation, but you will also be in better health yourself. You will remain healthier during pregnancy, make a faster recovery from the delivery, and be less likely to suffer from post-natal depression or premenstrual syndrome after the birth.

Becoming parents is an indescribable joy. Knowing that you have taken every possible step to ensure your baby's well-being can only enhance that joy.

Maryon Stewart,
Sussex, June 1995

CALLING ALL MUMS

Your Experiences Analysed

For many years now we have been told that smoking and drinking alcohol during pregnancy could damage an unborn child. There have been national health-education campaigns to get these messages across, which included graphic posters being hung in public places including many doctor and clinic waiting rooms. We have also been encouraged to eat a balanced diet and to take regular exercise during pregnancy. But have these campaigns really reached their target audience, and more importantly, have their messages been taken on board?

In order to assess how knowledgeable new mothers are about key health issues that relate to preconceptual care, pregnancy and weaning, we put together a survey which *First Steps* very kindly published in their magazine in February 1995, titled 'Calling All Mums'. You may have seen the survey, and if you actually took part in it, we are very grateful for your help. We were also very grateful for funds donated by both Sanatogen and Kimberly-Clark which allowed us to analyse the survey and arrive at conclusions which will help other health educators and hopefully tens of thousands of prospective mothers in the years to come.

The first part of the survey included a sample of 652 women who had had their last baby on average within the last five years. The average age of the women who participated was just under 28 years, and they had previously had an average of 1.5 children.

344 women (52.8%) had 1 child
212 women (32.5%) had 2 children
62 women (9.5%) had 3 children
25 women (3.8%) had 4 children
9 women (1.4%) had 5 children
2 women had 6 or more children, but were excluded from the analysis because the numbers in this group were too small.

I have not aimed to cover the subject of birth in this book as there are several excellent books which cover the pros and cons of different types of delivery. You will find details of these listed in the Appendix on page 275. However, we did ask about the type of delivery that our sample had experienced and the report was as below.

Survey of 652 Mothers (reporting for one or more births)
BIRTH METHODS

Water birth at home	None
Water birth in hospital	3 women
Home delivery	14 women
Caesarian section	127 women
Normal delivery in hospital	545 women
(22% of these had previously had a Caesarian section.)	

Only a small number of women had home confinements, and no-one had a home water birth. Having had one home delivery on 'dry land' myself, and two home water births (which I can thoroughly recommend), I was surprised by these figures.

We also asked our sample whether they had attended an ante-natal class, and again I found it surprising that 23 per cent of the women in the sample had not attended one though they had all probably attended an ante-natal clinic.

Survey of 652 Mothers
WHO ATTENDED ANTE-NATAL CLINIC/CLASSES

---

501 women (76.8%) attended an ante-natal class with their last pregnancy.

211 (32.3%) went to a class run by their health visitor
230 (35.2%) went to a class at their local hospital
28 (4.2%) went to classes run by the NCT
69 (13.8%) went to other classes

NB   Some women attended more than one class.

From the sample of 652 women we decided to concentrate our analysis on the 448 women who had given birth within fourteen months of completing the survey in February 1995. The reason for this was two-fold. Some of the answers to questions about what the mothers did before or during their pregnancy would be hard to remember for those whose babies were older. Secondly, all these mothers would have conceived after the advice given in December 1992 by the then Chief Medical Officer at the Department of Health for all women to take a supplement of folic acid (one of the B group of vitamins) prior to becoming pregnant. This was a turning point in the health care of future

7

babies and has helped to focus attention on the health and diet of women before pregnancy.

From the same survey we discovered that 23 per cent of the 448 women who had recently had a baby did not attend ante-natal classes, and a total of 10 per cent of these babies weighed less than 2.72 kg (6 lb). The average birth weight of babies born to first-time non-attenders was 3.2 kg (7 lb, 1½ oz) some 126 g (4½ oz) lighter than the babies of first-time mothers who attended ante-natal clinics. This, as you will discover, may be a key factor in determining the quality of health enjoyed by that child later on in life.

Whilst it was no surprise to me, I am sure it will make others stop in their tracks to realise that more women got educated about health during pregnancy from books and magazines than any other source. In fact the survey showed that more than three times more women *helped themselves* to information rather than seeking it from their doctor.

SOURCE OF HEALTH AND PREGNANCY INFORMATION

Source of Information	None	A Little	A Lot
Books	26	105	317
Magazines	27	140	281
Ante-natal Clinic	105	151	192
Mother/Female Relative	102	203	143
Doctor	74	274	100
Friends	115	236	97
Health Visitor	187	170	91
Television Programmes	195	205	48
Videos	317	104	27
Pharmacists	401	43	4
Other	402	29	17

* * *

70.8% (317 women) obtained their information mainly from books, and 62.7% (281 women) from magazines. Less than 50% of women received their information from ante-natal classes, just over 30% from their mother or a female relative, and only 22.3% obtained a lot of information from their doctor. Slightly less, 21.6%, were informed by friends, and a worrying 10.7% learned from television. Less than 1% received much information from their pharmacist.

Our survey examined other issues, including the type of diet followed before and during pregnancy, and social habits like smoking, alcohol consumption and the amount of tea and coffee consumed. We also looked at views on nutritional supplements before and during pregnancy, at exercise habits, and whether women were changing their habits in preparation for pregnancy. As you go through the book you will see that I have included our findings in the appropriate places.

What did shock us about the survey was that 46 per cent of the sample carried on either smoking or drinking in their preconceptual phase. Many cut down their consumption *during* pregnancy but this, as you will discover, was probably after the damage had been done. Additionally, 50 per cent of the sample did not make any attempt to eat either more fruit or more vegetables before becoming pregnant, and 4 per cent cut down their consumption of one or both before conceiving.

Any thoughts I may have had about retiring early have been laid to rest by the results of this survey. As you read through the information in Part One of this book you will realise that the health and well-being of the next generation is at stake if we do not make some crucial changes to our diet and lifestyle at least four months before we conceive a baby. There is no shortage of work to be done.

PART ONE
Healthy Parents

CHAPTER 1

Planning a Healthy Baby

Vets and zoo-keepers probably know more about producing healthy animal offspring than most doctors do about producing healthy humans, which is a sad state of affairs considering that we are approaching the end of the twentieth century. At a time when we build spaceships, send humans to the moon, build computers with the IQ of genius, only a minority of doctors are aware that the health of future generations lies in our hands today. Evidence exists to show that we can 'programme' the quality of health of unborn children by manipulating the diet and lifestyle of the prospective parents. However, instead of going from strength to strength, many of us are denying our children and *their* children the right to optimum health and intelligence in the long term, by largely ignoring the wealth of evidence to support the case for proper preconceptual planning.

It is estimated that some 30–40 per cent of babies born in the Western world are unplanned, which obviously means there was no healthy programme followed prior to conception. The majority of couples who *do* plan to conceive seem still to be pretty much in the dark about the dangers of inadequate planning. As both men and women may be exposed on a regular basis to agents which can cause birth defects, often before the woman knows that she is pregnant, making a pre-pregnancy plan is essential. Even prior to conception both your eggs and your partner's sperm are sensitive to their environment, and can easily be damaged. Whilst Mother Nature sometimes naturally terminates a pregnancy that is likely to have a poor outcome, the fertilised egg often goes on to become a live baby that is disadvantaged in some way, either physically or mentally, or both.

ENVIRONMENTAL FACTORS

The following environmental factors influence the health of a future pregnancy:

★ Alcohol, cigarettes, conventional drugs, illegal drugs, environmental toxins, e.g. pesticides, herbicides.
★ Lead from petrol and elsewhere, infections.
★ Deficiencies of vitamins, minerals and other essential nutrients.

These are factors both in men and women. In men sperm production is an on-going process taking about four months from the beginning of sperm production to its completion. In women, although only one egg is released per month, many are lying in waiting and begin a maturation process about 100 days prior to ovulation of that egg.

For both men and women, this three to four months' time prior to conception is the point at which environmental factors and dietary qualities seem to play a big part in determining the success and health of any future pregnancy.

From the time of conception, each minute bodily system has its own timetable for development, and the supply of essential nutrients and timing of contact with a toxin will determine the type of damage that results. The heart is formed between the third and sixth week, the limbs between the fourth and seventh week, and the palate between the sixth and eighth week. As the pregnancy progresses the brain and central nervous system develop, and the baby depends on a safe environment in order to thrive. Toxins can retard growth and development as well as influence intelligence and behaviour. Even the use of sedatives around the time of delivery, something which used to be recommended in hospitals, may result in a baby being lethargic at birth and at risk of developing respiratory problems.

According to recent American research data, babies who are undernourished in the first four weeks of development stand a much higher chance of developing heart disease, a major cause of death in middle age, and brain disorders, present from birth, which show up later in life in one in eight adults. In addition to this, for every child who has a diagnosed heart defect or brain disorder, there are others who have minor impairments which remain undiagnosed.

There are many factors that affect birth weight – among them smoking, the consumption of alcohol and certainly inadequate nutrition – and low birth weight remains one of the most serious public-health problems in the world today. A former co-ordinator of the World Health Organisation Maternal and Child Health Programme stated 'that more than twenty million low birth-weight babies are born every year ... they account for a high proportion of infant mortality. If they survive they suffer from higher rates of childhood illness and more or less permanent and severe disabling conditions such as mental retardation, behavioural disorders, cerebral palsy and impairment of vision and deafness.'

These are but a few of the 'invisible' pitfalls which make the difference between a normal healthy baby that lives a long healthy life, and a baby who at best has the appearance of being normal, but is plagued with poor health and limited intelligence throughout its relatively short life. When faced with the choice, all sane prospective parents would choose to have a healthy family. They would choose to be made fully aware of the pitfalls that are associated with inadequate preconceptual planning, and armed with the new knowledge would take every step to pre-empt them.

There is a wealth of published literature about the results of inadequate preconceptual planning, and the effects that our diet, social habits and indeed environment have on our unborn children. I find it hard to come to terms with the fact that all this information exists in books and in medical journals, but is not placed in the public domain for consumption, in lay terms, by the people who matter most, the prospective parents. If the information did not exist we could be forgiven for not taking responsibility for the consequences of our actions. But experts do now know a great deal about the secrets of a healthy life, and this book is my interpretation of their work, in simple terms, which will enable you to do all in your power to produce healthy children.

In this first part of the book I will take you through the effects that nutrition, social poisons and environmental factors have on the development of our growing children. I will then examine how both you and your partner can improve your fertility, the sort of preconceptual programme that you should be following, and details about the best time to conceive. I have also tried to answer many of the questions that you are likely to have. However, if any remain unanswered, or if you feel you need some personal help, the Women's Nutritional Advisory Service provides a service for individuals, details of which are on page 279.

I wish you well on your voyage of discovery and hope that the fruits of your knowledge bring you many years of happiness.

CHAPTER 2

The Effect of Nutrition on Birth Weight and Development

It is a somewhat daunting realisation that what we eat and how we live during the vital months before and during pregnancy will determine the quality of health and the length of time our children live. It places a great deal of responsibility on often young shoulders. There are so many ways in which we can influence the health prospects of our unborn children, and so many ways in which we can cause them damage without realising.

Babies born with a low birth weight below 2.5kgs (5.5lbs) are at an increased risk of developing heart disease, stroke, diabetes, high blood pressure and cholesterol levels in later life. Additionally, if organs are damaged or growth is impaired during the baby's development because of external factors, then that child may well suffer with other health problems. For example, if the lungs did not grow properly when in the womb, the child is likely later to suffer with chest infections, bronchitis and maybe asthma.

Infections in early infancy can also lead to other health problems in later life. People who have been susceptible to chest infections in childhood are likely candidates for bronchitis and pneumonia later on. If acute appendicitis occurs in adulthood, it may be linked to a gut infection acquired shortly after birth, which has been lying dormant.

It is important to understand how these major health

17

problems occur in the first place, and what we can do to circumvent them. Here are a few examples.

HEART DISEASE

Since the beginning of this century the incidence of coronary heart disease has been rapidly on the increase, making it the most common cause of death in the Western world. The rate at which this disease has been taking a grip on the population is too fast for its cause to be attributed to just genetic problems, so it must be something to do with our diet and lifestyle. Following the steep rise in prevalence, the last twenty years have seen a 25 per cent reduction in coronary heart disease in the USA, but not the UK, once again producing a trend that is too rapid to be associated with anything other than a change in nutrition and environmental factors during the developmental stages of a baby's life.

Nearly half a century of research into adult diet and lifestyle has provided only some of the answers. Cigarette smoking and our high consumption of animal fat have been targeted as the major reasons for the statistics taking a turn for the worse in the UK. Another confusing factor is that the incidence of coronary heart disease is higher in poorer areas of the country, and amongst lower income groups, groups that we now know tended to eat less well than the rest of the nation.

A large study in England and Wales, which examined almost one million deaths from coronary heart disease and pieced together the infant mortality records, made it possible to focus on the growing baby's early environment. This led researchers to look more closely at nutritional, hormonal and metabolic factors, and they then arrived at the theory that the health of the infant could be permanently 'programmed' during the crucial developmental stages. A simple example of these external factors involves the American alligator: if its eggs are incubated at a temperature of 30°C, all the offspring are female; at a temperature of 33°C, all the offspring are male. A temperature between the two produces offspring of both sexes. Such is the effect of the environment on development.

Two famous researchers, E. M. Widdowson and R. A. McCance, demonstrated that the timing of the inadequate environment was the all-important factor. They studied rats who were undernourished from the age of three to six weeks, just after their mother had finished feeding them. They lost weight and, despite being properly fed again from six weeks onwards, they failed to grow as expected and remained permanently small. A second group were denied adequate nutrition between the ages of nine to twelve weeks, but when they returned to a normal feeding routine, unlike the first group, they gained weight as expected. It is thought that at some time around the time of birth, growth rate is programmed according to resources. The first group of rats were obviously caught at a bad time and never recovered.

Numerous studies on animals show that if the mother is denied adequate protein or calories during pregnancy, she produces smaller offspring than would otherwise have been expected. The same is true for women. Curiously, women who eat less and less have smaller and smaller babies, whilst women who eat more have bigger babies, but reach a plateau after which the extra calories they consume do not seem to affect the size of the baby.

In 1966 the Medical Research Council discovered Herefordshire records that had been kept by a pioneer midwife, Miss Ethel Burnside, from 1911 until 1945. These records contained information about the birth weight of the baby, its weight at one year, plus details about weaning progress at one year, and the number of teeth present. The National

Health Service Register at Southport was used to trace 10,141 men born during 1911 and 1930, and 5,583 women born during 1923 and 1930. Tracing the female babies was much more difficult as many of them had married and changed their names. The study examined the health records of all those included and found, not surprisingly, that the low birth-weight babies, who remained small at the age of one, were most commonly the victims of coronary heart disease later in life.

HIGH BLOOD PRESSURE

It seems that high blood pressure is to some degree passed down from one generation to the next. Your baby's blood pressure is likely to reflect your own, which was more than likely passed to you from your mother.

It is common knowledge that people who are overweight tend to have higher blood pressure, but high blood pressure is also likely to occur in those that had a low birth weight, which is not widely appreciated. British studies in 1946 first suggested that blood pressure may be related to growth rate in the uterus before birth. Two major studies carried out in Sheffield and Preston both confirmed that high blood pressure was likely to present in those babies that were small for dates (in comparison to what they *should* be at that stage), rather than premature babies. These studies went on to show that the low birth-weight babies had different physical proportions to those babies whose weight was on target. The babies that were shorter and had a smaller abdominal circumference went on to have higher blood pressure in adult life. It would seem that poor growth before birth might mean a greater risk of high blood pressure in adult life.

You may be aware that table salt has also been linked to high blood pressure and consequently recommendations to adults to lower their salt intake are now standard. Whilst avoiding salt does tend to lower blood pressure to some degree, it is unlikely, however, to make up for the damage done prior to birth.

Another fascinating part of this picture is that babies who are small for dates, and likely to have high blood pressure later in life, have a different fingerprint pattern to normal weight babies. The patterns of the fingerprints are formed by approximately nineteen weeks. Both British and Indian studies have confirmed that babies who are born with a whorl on one or more finger are more likely to have high blood pressure later in life. Another physical sign is the shape of the palms of the hands. Babies who are short at birth in relation to the size of their head are likely to have narrow palms. Thus growth and development before birth are determining health in adult life.

DIABETES

Five studies have now shown that people who had low birth weight have increased chances of developing non-insulin dependent diabetes. Babies who are light for dates are seven times more likely to develop blood sugar problems or get diabetes than babies whose weight is in the normal range. Babies who are over 4.3 kg (9 lb, 9 oz) at birth are also at risk because their mother is herself more likely to have diabetes or a diabetic tendency during pregnancy.

The Preston study previously mentioned showed that babies who are both thin and short tend to be candidates for glucose impairment problems or diabetes. It was also discovered that placentas were heavier in relation to the birth weights of the babies, which suggests that they were undernourished during their development. Another study on infants who were small for dates has shown that they are likely to have less of the specialised cells in the pancreas that produce insulin, which are developing from the twelfth week of pregnancy right through to the fifth month of life.

Gaining excessive weight in adult life may put a strain on blood sugar control that the underweight baby is ill-equipped to deal with. Some researchers feel that an undernourished developing baby learns to be thrifty with nutrients and for as long as it remains undernourished its blood sugar control remains adequate. An improvement in nutritional state in adult life may well be the factor that shows up the deficiency of the specialised insulin producing cells, resulting in diabetes. Other factors like smoking, the ageing process and physical inactivity later in life may also be enough to trigger the disease. Low birth weight would seem to be a 'marker' for those at risk of diabetes in later life.

CHRONIC BRONCHITIS

Until relatively recently it was accepted that chronic bronchitis and other chest infections were mainly due to environmental factors such as smoking, air temperature and geographical location. More recent research has shown that these factors are only part of the story. Impaired lung growth during the developmental stages and early infant life, due to inadequate nutrition and environmental conditions, point to potential abnormal lung function and disease in adult life.

The lungs of male and female babies develop at different stages and end up having different dimensions. Boys have larger lungs with narrower airways, which take longer to develop. It seems that boys have more problems with chest infections in infancy than girls, and are more likely to need treatment, probably due to that size difference. But it is not all bad news, as breast-feeding is a recognised way of reducing the number of chest infections that your children suffer.

Recent research suggests that the disproportionately short baby, who fails to grow at the optimum rate during infancy, is more likely to develop chronic bronchitis as the years go by. Being below average weight at the age of one also seems to be an indication of predisposition to chest problems. Another study suggests that our lung function is 'programmed' during the developing months in the uterus, making those whose lungs are impaired from the start more susceptible to chronic chest complaints in later life.

There is enough new evidence to convince even the most sceptical amongst us that diet and environmental factors, from the time of conception until the child is well into the first year of life, have the power to programme the health of that child for a lifetime. With that in mind, let us now move on to examine the many ways that you can improve your chances of having a healthy bouncing baby.

CHAPTER 3

Essential Nutrients for You and Your Baby

A healthy diet has to provide an adequate supply of energy and protein, which are necessary for building tissues – and essential vitamins, minerals and specialised fats called essential fatty acids. The majority of energy comes from fats and carbohydrates, and a small amount from protein-rich foods in our diet.

PROTEIN

Protein is a general term given to a series of complex chemicals that are widely found in many foods which we associate with being nutritious. They are composed of individual amino acids (essential building blocks to structure ourselves), many hormones, enzymes and other agents involved in the intricate metabolism of living organisms. If protein intake is not adequate in the diet, then tissue growth and repair cannot take place and we break down our own protein-rich tissues, especially muscle. Increased protein intake is required during pregnancy, not only for the growth of the baby, but also for the growth of other protein-rich tissues including the extra blood cells, of the uterus in particular, and the placenta. Protein can be found from both animal sources – meats, eggs, dairy products including milk and cheese – and vegetarian sources, especially peas, beans, lentils, nuts, seeds and, to a very small extent, rice and potatoes. It is always a good idea to have a wide variety of protein sources, especially if you are vegetarian or semi-vegetarian. Protein deficiency is rare outside of Third World countries, but there is increasing concern that protein intakes may only just be adequate in many cash-poor vegetarians in the UK. This could affect the growth and development of your baby.

FATS

Fats are predominantly a source of energy. There are a wide variety of different fats which are all chemically similar, and all provide a rich source of energy, 9 kilocalories per gramme weight over twice the energy content of same weight of carbohydrate or sugar. The chemical structure of fats varies, depending upon the source – either animal or vegetable. Most vegetable fats are liquid at room temperature, i.e. are usually oils. Many are polyunsaturates and contain specialised essential fatty acids which are used not only as sources of calories, but help in the building of the structure of the cells, especially those of the skin and nervous system. Most animal fats are rich saturated fats which serve only as a source of calories. Excessive intake of saturated fats, and lack of fibre, vitamins and minerals in the diet, may predispose to heart disease. Our own bodies store excess calories from whatever source as fats.

CARBOHYDRATES

These come in various forms, and all are based around the structure of simple sugars. Starch is a complicated amalgam of many different sugars which are broken down into individual sugars by our digestive processes. Starchy foods include all cereals, potatoes, rice and root vegetables. All simple sugars are found in milk, table sugar, honey and fruit. Though chemically similar, they may have different properties for health. For example, high intakes of sucrose, table sugar, predisposes particularly to dental caries or tooth decay. All, however, can be regarded as simple energy. Often in their natural state, i.e. fruits and vegetables, these sugar and starch-rich foods are also rich in the vitamins and minerals necessary for sugar metabolism, especially Vitamin B and magnesium. Refined foods such as cakes, biscuits and sweets have been processed in such a way that these essential vitamins and minerals are lost and have to be found from other parts of the diet.

FIBRE

Fibre is also a type of carbohydrate which, by definition, is not digested. It mainly comes from the cell walls of plants – cellulose – and is resistant to our digestive processes. Because of its water-resistant properties, it forms the bulk of our stool. A high-fibre diet is a diet rich in fruit, vegetables and cereals, which brings with it many nutritional benefits, for example, lowering the blood cholesterol and with that a lower risk of heart disease. Excessive consumption of fibre-rich foods, especially bran, may inhibit the absorption of certain essential nutrients including calcium and other minerals. It is best to eat a wide variety of fibre-rich foods, especially fresh fruits and vegetables.

VITAMINS

Vitamins are unlike protein, fats and carbohydrates in that they are required in minute quantities. They are not a source of energy, but are required by the energy-releasing chemical reactions in the body. A deficiency of them results in disturbance of the metabolism, producing a variety of distinctive symptoms and signs. They each play a crucial role in growth and development. In principle, deficiency before conception and during the early stages of pregnancy is likely to influence the outcome of pregnancy. However, the exact function in human pregnancy is not well identified, mainly because one cannot conduct experiments in humans in the way that one can in rats and mice!

VITAMIN A

This is necessary for growth and development. It plays an essential role in the working of the retina at the back of the eye. Vitamin A comes in two forms: retinol is animal-derived, and beta-carotene derives from plant sources. The World Health Organisation recommends that women consume 800 mcg of Vitamin A per day, increasing to 1,000 during pregnancy. Good sources of retinol are liver, oily fish, dairy products like milk, cheese, yoghurt and butter, plus eggs, kidneys and margarine (which is fortified with Vitamin A as retinol). An excess of Vitamin A as retinol can be dangerous, though, and is associated with congenital birth defects. Women are warned not to take supplements of Vitamin A as retinol without their doctor's recommendation, and not to eat liver whilst pregnant or breast-feeding. Due to over-fortification of animal feeds, the Vitamin A content of many animals' livers has trebled since 1980.

Beta-carotene is the plant form of the vitamin, which does not build up in the body. It is a powerful antioxidant, which protects against cell damage from environmental poisons, and is necessary for maintaining a healthy immune system. It could help reduce the toxic effect of environmental chemicals in babies and adults. Whilst the UK does not have a recommended intake of beta-carotene, the National Cancer

Institute in the USA recommends that adults consume 6 mg per day in order to reduce the risk of cancer. Foods rich in beta-carotene are dark green vegetables and yellow fruits and vegetables.

B VITAMINS

This is a family of several vitamins with similar or related properties.

VITAMIN B1

This vitamin, also known as thiamin, is essential for foetal growth, especially crucial to the development of the nervous system. It is necessary for energy production from carbo-hydrates and the manufacture of some of the important amino acids.

The recommended daily intake is 0.8 mg. In the UK it is suggested that pregnant women should increase their intake of thiamin by 0.1 mg during pregnancy and 0.2 mg whilst breast-feeding. Many cereals are fortified with thiamin, and it can also be found in wheatgerm, whole-grain products, pota-toes, cornflakes, Brazil nuts, pulses, meat and seafood. Excess alcohol destroys thiamin, and those eating large amounts of convenience foods for a long period may become deficient.

VITAMIN B2

Also known as riboflavin, this is essential as well for the production of energy and for carbohydrate metabolism. The requirement for adult women is 1.1 mg with an increase of 0.3 mg in pregnancy and 0.5 mg during lactation. You will find it in milk, cheese, yoghurt, cereals, meat, green leafy vegetables and fruit.

VITAMIN B3

Otherwise known as niacin, B3 is particularly important for normal metabolic function and energy production. The UK recommendations are 13 mg per day for an adult, with an additional 2 mg during breast-feeding. Rich sources of niacin are cereals, meat, poultry, fish, and nuts.

VITAMIN B5
Better known as pantothenic acid, B5 is essential for normal metabolism of carbohydrates, protein and fats. It is commonly found in many of the health foods listed so far, so whilst eating a healthy diet it is almost impossible to become deficient.

VITAMIN B6
Also called pyridoxine, this vitamin plays a particularly important role in rapid cell division, the production of red blood cells and the development of the foetus. It is also needed for proper enzyme function. The UK Reference Nutrient Intake is 1.2 mg with no additional amount during pregnancy and breast-feeding.

You will find Vitamin B6 in cereals, whole-grain products, wheatgerm, soya, bananas, meat, beans and nuts. If you have been taking large doses of Vitamin B6 to keep your premenstrual syndrome at bay you will need to reduce these during the preconceptual phase, and replace them with a lower dose supplement.

VITAMIN B12
Known also as cobalamin, B12 is vital for the production of the genetic material called DNA, which is constantly being produced during the growth of your baby. It works in conjunction with folic acid, and deficiency can result in abnormally large cells. Adequate levels of Vitamin B12 are now acknowledged as being important for the prevention of neural tube defects (or spina bifida). Recent research has shown that women with low levels of B12 are five times more likely to have a baby with neural tube defect, so it is recommended that supplements are taken during the pre-

conceptual phase right through to at least the end of the first three months of pregnancy.

The UK currently only recommends 1.5 mcg per day rising to 2 mcg per day during breast-feeding, whilst other countries recommend levels of up to 3 mcg. However, this may change in the near future as a result of the new research. Most meat-eating women consume about 5 mcg per day, but vegetarians and particularly vegans are at risk of deficiency, and many should be taking supplements from preconception to the end of breast-feeding.

FOLIC ACID

This B vitamin, together with Vitamin B12, plays a crucial role in the prevention of neural tube defect, spina bifida, in the growing foetus. It is also necessary for the formation of red blood cells and genetic material.

The neural tube is a cylinder of tissue, derived initially from the skin of a baby, which goes on to form the spine and brain. Two neural tube defects have been strongly linked with poor intakes of folic acid. They are spina bifida and anencephaly. Spina bifida is where the tissues that will form the nerves of the spine fail to fold in on themselves as they develop, thus usually leaving the lower end of the spine undeveloped. This may be obvious at birth as a swelling, or even exposed tissue, which leads to poor function of the nerves to the legs. Difficulties in walking, and bladder and bowel difficulties as a result of nerve damage, may then be present throughout childhood and adult life. In anencephaly, the other end of the neural tube, which would go on to form the brain, fails to form. This may lead to death of the baby before birth or shortly after. The growth and development of this nervous tissue is very dependent upon an adequate supply of folic acid. The absence of folic acid in the mother's diet can lead to either of these two neural tube defects.

It is estimated that over 70 per cent of neural tube defects can be prevented by taking folic acid, also known as folate. To reduce the risk of spina bifida, the amount of folic acid required during the preconceptual phase and the first three months of pregnancy is at least *double* the usual requirement. It can be found in green leafy vegetables, and in fact was first discovered in spinach. Other good sources are cereals, chick peas, meat, oranges and orange juice, potatoes, asparagus, sweetcorn and milk.

The recommendation from the Chief Medical Officer in the UK in December 1992 was that all women planning to conceive should take a daily supplement of 0.4mg (400 mcg) prior to conception, until the end of the third month of pregnancy. Women who have given birth already to a child with spina bifida should be given a supplement of 4 mg (4,000 mcg) per day by their doctor.

Sadly our survey of new mothers showed that large numbers of women who had recently had a baby didn't even know about folic acid, and many of those that did were confused. We analysed the attitudes of two groups of women, those that had babies before the directive was issued in 1992, and those that had had their babies more recently.

Survey of 448 Mothers
ATTITUDES TO FOLIC ACID

Those who had given birth in the last 5 months were asked about their attitudes to folic acid before the pregnancy.

34.8% did not know about it

28.8% thought it could be taken at any time before pregnancy

25.8% thought it should be taken only in the first three months of the pregnancy

15.1% thought it should be taken once pregnant

13.1% thought it was not needed if on a balanced diet
8.1% thought it should be taken throughout the pregnancy
5.6% thought it should be taken if suggested by the ante-natal clinic
7.1% thought it should be taken a year before pregnancy

The same questions were put to a second group, women whose babies were older than 6 months and up to 14 months.

43.2% did not know about it
21.6% thought it could be taken at any time before pregnancy
25.2% thought it should be taken only in the first three months of the pregnancy
14% thought it should be taken once pregnant
12.8% didn't think it was needed if on a balanced diet
12% thought it should be taken during the whole pregnancy
4% thought it should be taken if suggested by the ante-natal clinic
5.2% thought it should be taken a year before pregnancy

The number of women who had heard of the vitamin and its significance had improved in this first group, but there was still a great deal of confusion about its value and when it should be taken.

VITAMIN C
This water-soluble vitamin promotes wound healing, prevents scurvy, and is necessary for the production of collagen, the structural protein of our bodies. It is also an antioxidant, which gobbles up free radicals – chemicals that can potentially damage foetal growth. It is particularly valuable in aiding iron absorption from vegetarian sources. It is also thought to increase sperm motility at a dose of 250 mg per day or more.

Recommendations for daily amounts of Vitamin C vary from country to country, ranging from 80 mg in the Netherlands to 40 mg in the UK. Most fruits and vegetables contain Vitamin C, particularly citrus fruits, blackcurrants, mangoes and strawberries, and potatoes, broccoli, Brussels sprouts and apple juice. It is important to know, however, that this vitamin is destroyed by boiling. Vegetables should therefore either be eaten raw, or steamed or very lightly cooked in order to preserve as much of the nutrients as possible. Many finger foods, which can be eaten by older babies, contain substantial amounts of Vitamin C, like fruit for example.

VITAMIN D

This vitamin is mainly synthesised through the skin from sunlight. It is needed for healthy bones and teeth, and to help the absorption of calcium. It is present in only a few fortified foods, oily fish like mackerel, sardines, herring and salmon, and eggs to a lesser extent. A deficiency may result in impaired brain development of a foetus, an abnormally shaped skull and possible learning difficulties, so mothers are now advised to take Vitamin D during pregnancy, in order to pass on adequate stores to the growing baby.

Breast-milk only contains small amounts of Vitamin D, so you will need to eat plenty of oily fish, get your baby out into the daylight whenever possible, and give supplements to babies over six months of age. Pregnant Asian and West Indian women and their children are particularly at risk of Vitamin D deficiency because of poorer production of Vitamin D in darker skin. Lack of sunlight exposure in city dwellers is still a significant risk factor today.

VITAMIN E

This is another antioxidant vitamin, whose function is to mop up the free radicals that damage our cells. It is also needed for healthy sperm, and in fact trials are currently being done on Vitamin E and male infertility.

Although present European dietary recommendations for Vitamin E are only 10 mg per day, many experts believe that a daily intake of at least 40–50 mg is needed to protect against the free radical damage that can result in heart disease. Supplements of natural Vitamin E may be taken by pregnant women, and will ensure the baby receives adequate stores.

Vitamin E can be found in wheatgerm oil, oily fish, nuts, vegetable oils like sunflower (and the seeds), cod liver oil and milk. Babies born with inadequate reserves of Vitamin E usually have fragile red blood cell membranes, and are often jaundiced. Poor development of the brain and other major organs, and developmental difficulties often follow.

Survey of 448 New Mothers
USAGE OF SUPPLEMENTS PRIOR TO PREGNANCY

	Group I Baby born 0–5 months ago 198 women			Group II Baby born 6–14 months ago 250 women		
	Never	*Occa-sionally*	*Regu-larly*	*Never*	*Occa-sionally*	*Regu-larly*
Iron	74.2%	15.2%	10.6%	71.6%	14.8%	13.6%
Folic acid	65.2%	8.1%	26.8%	70.8%	8.0%	21.2%
Multi-Vitamins	65.6%	22.7%	11.6%	58.4%	22.4%	19.2%
Vitamin B	92.4%	5.6%	2.0%	88.8%	8.0%	3.2%
Evening Primrose Oil	90.8%	5.6%	3.6%	90.4%	5.6%	4.0%

MINERALS

Minerals can be divided into two types. One type are the bulk minerals required for the structure of tissues and cells, especially the skeleton and teeth, and these include calcium, phosphorus, magnesium, sodium and potassium. The other type are trace elements which function like vitamins, enhancing essential metabolic and chemical reactions in the body. Some of the bulk minerals, especially calcium and magnesium, function in this manner as well.

Let us examine the role of each mineral, and see how much we need to consume per day.

CALCIUM

This is necessary for the development of strong bones and teeth, and it is mainly present in the skeleton. It is also needed for the smooth functioning of the immune system, and for muscle function, nerve conduction and blood coagulation. Babies born to mothers with low calcium levels tend to be smaller at birth and are slower to develop. A mother with low calcium levels stands a good chance of developing the bone-thinning disease, osteoporosis, as calcium will automatically be shifted from her bones and transferred to her growing baby.

The Reference Nutrient Intake, a safe level recommended by the Department of Health, at the moment in the UK is only 700 mg, with an additional 550 mg recommended during breast-feeding. The American National Institute of Health has recommended that older women increase their calcium intake to 1,500 mg per day in order to eliminate the risk of osteoporosis. In the UK, the National Osteoporosis Society is suggesting that the Government increase their recommendations so that pregnant and nursing mothers are instructed to take 1,200 mg per day, and pregnant and nursing teenagers 1,500 mg per day.

You will find plenty of calcium in milk of all types. Yoghurt, cheese, whole grains, soya products, sardines, sprats, whitebait, almonds and spinach also contain good amounts.

You can get much of the calcium you need just by drinking

an extra pint of milk per day. Calcium supplements are widely available, but some of them do not dissolve fully in the gut. Do not take calcium supplements with bran or bran containing foods as the phytic acid in the bran reduces the absorption of calcium

CHROMIUM

A minute quantity of this important mineral is present in a high concentration in our body at birth. It is vital for the normal function of the hormone insulin. A lack of chromium is associated with poor blood sugar control, and thus may contribute to diabetes in later life. The UK does not have a RNI (Reference Nutrient Intake) for chromium, but the National Research Council in the USA suggests between 50 and 200 mcg per day for an adult. Supplements are available, but often only small amounts are absorbed.

Chromium-rich food are brewer's yeast, chilli peppers, green peppers, chicken, whole grains and potatoes. Black pepper is also an excellent source, and a good way of ensuring you get an adequate daily amount.

COPPER

Small amounts of copper are needed for brain chemical metabolism and for the healthy functioning of major organs like the liver and brain, and the muscles. In the developing baby it is needed for all tissue growth. Babies born near to or after their due date are likely to have enough copper stores to last them for four months. The premature baby, however, is at risk of deficiency.

The amount of copper needed per day is thought to be approximately 1.5 mg, and its content in food varies, depending on the copper content of the soil in which it was grown. Good sources are shellfish, green vegetables, dried fruits, beans and peas. Breast-milk is a good source of copper, but its concentration dwindles at around four months.

Copper supplements should not be taken without expert advice as they may displace zinc and iron.

IODINE

This is necessary for the development of the central nervous system and for the production of thyroid hormones. Most of the iodine we consume comes from milk, both breast- and cow's, and a deficiency is rare since the introduction of iodised salt in the UK. However, in underdeveloped countries, iodine deficiency still occurs, and mothers still risk giving birth to babies with cretinism.

IRON

Iron deficiency is the most commonly reported world-wide, and women of child-bearing age are the group most at risk. Iron is essential for the production of red blood cells and deficiency can result in anaemia. Iron-deficient children are reported to have poor growth and development, be less intelligent, and to have poorer appetites and less energy. Three months' treatment with iron supplements may correct the problems associated with deficiency, if given at the appropriate time of development. There are suggestions that if left too late, the developmental problems cannot be fully reversed.

During pregnancy the amount of red blood cells increases by some 30 per cent. Although the mother will be saving iron by not having periods, she will still need to take an iron-rich diet and perhaps consider taking supplements, especially in the latter half of pregnancy and whilst breast-feeding. In the UK the Reference Nutrient Intake for women is 14.8 mg, with no recommended increase for pregnancy. In the USA the recommendations double for pregnancy from 15 to 30 mg per day. If you have a history of heavy periods you are much more likely to need iron supplements, and 10 per cent of menstruating women are unable to satisfy their iron needs by diet alone.

Babies who are born roughly on time accumulate stores of iron in their liver. However, premature babies miss out on this, and are particularly at risk of deficiency during the first year of their lives. Human milk only contains small quantities of iron, although in an easily absorbable form, thus the baby is protected for approximately the first four months of life, after which it needs to be supplemented by the diet (you can get some tips about improving iron absorption on page 157). Good sources of iron are green leafy vegetables, meat, beans, fortified cereals and eggs.

MAGNESIUM
Magnesium is the most commonly deficient nutrient amongst women with premenstrual syndrome, with 50 per cent having mildly reduced levels in their red blood cells. Magnesium is needed for brain chemical metabolism, normal hormone function, smooth muscle control and the release of energy from carbohydrates. A lack of magnesium during pregnancy may lead to higher blood pressure, premature labour, painful unco-ordinated contractions during labour, and possibly miscarriage.

There are no obvious signs of magnesium deficiency, but muscle cramps, constipation, fatigue, insomnia and poor appetite are all associated with inadequate magnesium intake.

The Reference Nutrient Intake in the UK for women is 270 mg per day with an extra 50 mg whilst breast-feeding. Rich sources of magnesium are green leafy vegetables, nuts, seafood, soya products, whole grains, beans, meat, eggs and milk. If you are considering taking a supplement, an easily absorbable form of magnesium is amino acid chelate.

MANGANESE
Another antioxidant which is necessary for normal brain chemical metabolism and the brain chemical, dopamine.

Lack of manganese has been associated with infertility, poor foetal growth, birth defects and still-born animals.

There is no Reference Nutrient Intake for manganese in the UK, but observations show that pregnant women consume approximately 5.5 mg per day, with some 4 mg being lost in waste products. Rich sources of manganese, again depending on the soil used to grow the food, are whole grains, nuts, seeds, yeast, green leafy vegetables, fruit and eggs.

PHOSPHORUS

Most phosphorus in the body is linked to the calcium in our bones and teeth. It is needed for normal metabolism and energy release in particular. Phosphorus is widely available in our diet, and deficiency is rare other than in the alcoholic.

POTASSIUM

Potassium is of major importance in the transmission of messages from our brain, for normal muscle contraction and blood pressure, and for keeping our body fluids in balance. The richest sources are fruit, vegetables, beans, peas, meat, nuts and seeds.

SELENIUM

Although only needed in small amounts, selenium is a powerful antioxidant that works in conjunction with Vitamins A, C and E to protect us from cell damage. It is also needed for cell growth and the warding off of infection.

The UK Reference Nutrient Intake for selenium is 60 mcg per day, with an additional 15 mcg recommended for the breast-feeding period. Selenium in excess can be toxic.

Selenium-rich foods include whole grains, wheatgerm, nuts, yeast, broccoli, cabbage, onions, garlic, meat, fish, celery and mushrooms.

ZINC

Zinc is needed for growth and development, for normal immune function and for maintaining the structure of genetic material. Zinc is necessary for normal sperm count, which is not surprising as about 2 mg of zinc are lost with each ejaculation.

Good dietary sources are all protein-rich foods of animal or vegetable origin, including meat, milk, whole-grain products, nuts, cheese, yeast, seafood and eggs.

The absorption of zinc from food can be reduced, as can that of iron, by the presence of phytic acid which is found in bran and to a lesser extent wholemeal bread. The message is that you should not consume these to excess. Poor intake of zinc by the mother is associated with low birth weight, reduced length and head circumference. Giving supplements during pregnancy has little or no effect on these measures, but correcting a lack before conception may well be effective.

New European guidelines suggest that we should be taking 15 mg of zinc per day, and the observed average is about a third less than that. As far as infants are concerned, a Ministry of Agriculture, Fisheries and Foods survey in 1986 showed that 6 per cent of infants had daily zinc intakes which were below an acceptable level. Although much zinc comes from milk sources, meat and meat products are the richest source of zinc, and the recommendation of this survey was that we should offer our children larger servings of meat.

Case History

Rowena already had two children, and was no stranger to the medical profession. After her first pregnancy, her thyroid gland began to swell and then required removal because of early cancerous change. Since then she needs supplements of thyroid hormone, Vitamin D and calcium. She had attended our clinic because of her concerns about her diet now that she was five months' pregnant.

Her diet was in fact quite good, with significant regular intakes of fresh fruit, vegetables, fish and chicken. Overall her protein intake was only just satisfactory. However, a blood test showed a reduced level of magnesium and an exceptionally low level of zinc – about half the lower end of normal. Deficiency of this degree is strongly associated with growth problems. In addition to her iron and folic acid supplement, she began to take modest supplements of magnesium and zinc which she continued through to the end of the (successful) pregnancy.

The cause of her low zinc was never fully ascertained. It was corrected by her eating more zinc- and protein-rich foods and by her taking supplements.

ESSENTIAL FATTY ACIDS

The essential fatty acids, or EFAs, are long-chain polyunsaturated fatty acids which especially during the last three months of pregnancy, are crucial for growth and development of the baby, and in particular its central nervous system. Relatively recent evidence suggests that a deficiency of these long-chain polyunsaturated fatty acids in the tissues of developing babies results in low birth weight, which may have a life-long impact.

During pregnancy the essential fatty acid requirements of the infant are supplied via the placenta from the mother's stores and, once born, from breast-milk which contains high concentrations of essential fatty acids as opposed to formula milk. However, it seems that even babies born after an apparently normal pregnancy may have a borderline essential fatty acid status. Premature babies have a limited capacity to synthesise the long-chain polyunsaturated fatty acids from the mother's diet, which is a tricky situation because the brain grows very rapidly from the twenty-fifth week of pregnancy right through to the first few months after birth.

Good sources of the relevant fatty acids can be found in almonds, walnuts, hazelnuts, safflower and other seeds and their oils, eggs, fatty fish like salmon, mackerel and herring, turkey and lean game meats. The two types of essential fatty acids are linoleic acid and alpha-linolenic acid which respectively give rise to families of fats known as Omega 6 and Omega 3. They have a variety of functions, influencing the structure of many cells, especially in the nervous system, the immune system and our skin, and controlling inflammation in the body. Some people may not be good at converting these EFAs into their active forms. This requires a good diet, plenty of Vitamins B and C, and zinc, and is disrupted by alcohol and smoking.

Evening primrose oil contains gamma-linolenic acid. This essential fatty acid from the Omega 6 series is rapidly converted in the body into the two long-chain essential fatty acids which are most important to the health of the new-born infant. Marine fish oil, such as cod liver oil, provides Omega 3 essential fatty acids which are particularly important for the development of the brain and the eye.

Adequate intake of EFAs in the new-born infant seem to influence vision and subsequent intelligence. This may well explain why some breast-fed infants make better progress than bottle-fed ones. Ensuring a good dietary intake of EFAs in the mother's diet during the pregnancy may be vital to the baby's development. Supplements of EFAs may prove to be needed by some pregnant women, and indeed in Japan, Snow Brand, their most popular infant formula, contains Efamol evening primrose oil. Milupa in Germany also add evening primrose oil, and it seems that other baby milk manufacturers are contemplating it.

Trials feeding Efamol Marine – a combination of evening primrose and marine fish oils – to pregnant women during the final three months of pregnancy are on-going. Another study on breast-feeding mothers using Efamol evening primrose oil from between two to eight months of feeding, showed improved levels of essential fatty acids at a time when the natural supply in the milk would be tailing off. Because this oil contains only fatty acids which form a normal part of the diet, and because it is produced to high standards of quality control, it has been demonstrated to be a safe supplement. Efamol evening primrose oil and Efamol Marine are available in most chemists. The recommended dose is in the region of 2 g per day for those women whose diets are poor or low in these oils during the last three months of pregnancy.

SIMPLE DIETARY RECOMMENDATIONS FOR PRE-CONCEPTION

Here are some simple recommendations which, if you follow them, will help achieve an adequate intake of all the essential nutrients we have discussed. This is especially important in the preconceptual phase and in the first weeks of pregnancy as it determines the growth and development of your baby.

★ Eat three regular meals a day. Doing so will give you the best chance of obtaining a balanced intake of all essential nutrients. Do not miss meals.
★ Eat a cooked main meal per day. Cooked meat, fish or vegetarian based meals will again allow a good intake of essential nutrients, especially protein.
★ Eat at least one portion (120 g / 4 oz) of meat or fish or vegetarian protein, such as beans, peas or lentils. Many convenience or prepared meals are low in protein, vitamins and minerals.

43

★ Ensure a good intake of foods rich in folic acid, especially green leafy vegetables, fortified breakfast cereals, oranges and orange juice, eggs, almonds, and sweetcorn. You can eat liver once or twice a month if you so wish.

★ Enjoy good sources of calcium, including dairy products, milk (whole, skimmed or semi-skimmed) and cheese, but avoid soft cheese and cottage cheese. Soft cheese may contain the infecting organism Listeria (see page 120), and cottage cheese is low in protein and B vitamins.

★ Eat at least three portions of fruit per day, and two portions of green vegetables or green salad per day. This is in line with the latest recommendations for healthy eating for the general population, and will help maintain a good intake of fibre, vitamins and minerals.

★ Eat two or three slices of wholemeal bread per day. White bread may be acceptable if the rest of the diet is well balanced. Some will need more bread than others, and those on weight-reducing diets may need to consume less.

★ Use good quality vegetable oils, which are rich in essential fatty acids, especially sunflower, safflower, grapeseed and walnut. Olive oil is not rich in essential fatty acids. Use margarines based on these oils, e.g. sunflower margarine oil, or you can use a small amount of butter. Again, cut down on these if you need to lose weight.

★ Eat from a selection of other foods rich in essential fatty acids. These include oily fish, mackerel, herring and, to a lesser extent, salmon, spinach, walnuts, almonds, hazelnuts and pecans (peanuts are not so nutritious in this respect), and beans, especially pinto beans.

★ Trim the skin and fat from meat and poultry. These foods tend to be high in the less helpful saturated fats, and most of the environmental toxins, if present, will be found in the fatty portions of these foods.

★ Do not consume any alcohol. This is probably the best advice, though it is obviously hard for someone to follow.

Especially do not drink from about day 10 of your cycle until when your period begins, when your egg is at its most vulnerable.

★ Do not smoke or, if this is difficult, cut down. As you will see, there are many adverse affects of smoking on pregnancy.
★ Get your partner to follow the same dietary recommendations. The health of the father-to-be can also be a factor in the health of your future offspring.

If for some reason you are unable to follow these dietary recommendations, due to underlying medical conditions, allergy to a food or time restraints, then consider taking an appropriate nutritional supplement. Smokers, those consuming alcohol, and those with a poor intake of fresh fruit and vegetables, should consider taking an appropriate multivitamin and mineral supplement designed for the preconceptual time (see below). Those with a low intake of dairy products should probably have a calcium supplement unless consuming significant amounts of calcium-fortified soya milk and other calcium-rich foods. Those with medical problems requiring drug treatment may require specialist advice.

Survey of 448 Mothers
BEFORE YOUR LAST PREGNANCY DID YOU CHANGE
YOUR CONSUMPTION OF:

	No reply	More	Less	Stopped	No change	Never consumed
(All did not know value of folic acid)						
Fresh fruit	11	172	9	0	248	8
Fresh vegetables	11	134	8	1	290	14

Alcohol	10	3	112	155	64	104
Cigarettes	12	6	46	56	48	280
Sugar/sweets	10	62	120	4	240	12
Meat	11	45	34	1	325	32
Tea/coffee	10	30	144	22	221	21

The results of this section of the survey showed that the healthy eating message was getting across to some of the women, but by no means all of them. 38 per cent did start eating more fruit before their last pregnancy, and 30 per cent ate more fresh vegetables. 35 per cent of the sample stopped drinking alcohol, with a further 25 per cent reducing their consumption.

33 per cent of our sample who smoked stopped smoking before their last pregnancy and a further 27 per cent reduced their consumption. However, on the down side, 32 per cent of the smokers continued to smoke the same or more during their preconceptual phase, 15 per cent did not change or increased their alcohol consumption and 14 per cent ate more sugar and sweet food at this vital time.

NUTRITIONAL SUPPLEMENTS IN THE PRECONCEPTUAL PHASE AND DURING PREGNANCY

Multi-vitamins
Many multi-vitamins from chemists are not suitable as they will contain animal Vitamin A (retinol) and inadequate amounts of folic acid (i.e. not enough to prevent neural tube defects). The majority of these should not be taken during the preconceptual phase.

Pronatal
This specialist multi-vitamin and mineral supplement contains Vitamin A as beta-carotene, and good amounts of

folic acid, B vitamins and some minerals. It has a long record of safety and success with European women in the pre-conceptual phase and during the early part of pregnancy and breast-feeding. It is suitable for those with poor or uncertain dietary intakes, smokers and those still drinking alcohol.

Another product made by Blackmores called Specifics For Women which contains 500 mcg's of folic acid is available in Australia and New Zealand.

Pregnavite-Forte
This is an NHS prescribable multi-vitamin and mineral supplement, and is especially useful for those women who have given birth to a child with a neural tube defect. Again, it has a proven track record of prevention and safety.

Folic Acid
A 400 mcg strength, now widely available, is recommended to be taken by all women prior to conception. This dosage is now being incorporated into many multi-vitamin and other preparations.

4 mg is recommended for those women who have already given birth to a child with a neural tube defect and wish to conceive again.

Vitamin B12
Supplements ranging in dosage from 5 to 20 mcg are available in tablet form or usually combined with Vitamin B or multi-vitamin preparations. Vitamin B12 supplements should be taken by all women who are vegan, especially of longer than four years' duration. Vegetarians who consume no eggs and little in the way of dairy produce should also consider taking Vitamin B12 alone or in combination with other B vitamins.

Calcium
Doses of 500–1,000 mg may be required as supplements for those who are on a dairy-free diet or otherwise consuming foods low in calcium. Women from inner-city communities, especially dark-skinned women, may need additional calcium and Vitamin D supplements. The latter should provide 400 iu (international units) or 10mcg per day.

Cod Liver Oil
Most forms of cod liver oil in supplement form should not be taken prior to conception as they contain Vitamin A as retinol. They were once recommended as a source of Vitamin D for urban-dwelling, dark-skinned women during pregnancy and breast-feeding. Other sources of Vitamin D with calcium are preferred.

Magnesium
Supplements of magnesium may be useful for women with premenstrual syndrome. Doses can be safely taken in pregnancy if needed. The usual dose is 200–300 mg per day.

Zinc
Zinc supplements of approximately 10–15 mg a day may be needed by some women on a restricted diet, those with serious digestive problems and also men! Correction of zinc deficiency in men can help improve sperm count. Seek specialist advice.

Evening Primrose Oil
Evening primrose oil contains the specialised essential fatty acid, GLA. This is known to help premenstrual breast tenderness and eczema, and women with these problems should consider a supplement of 2–3 g of EPO per day, as Efamal. Some forms can be prescribed under the National Health.

Fish Oil Preparations
In addition to cod liver oil, other marine oil preparations are becoming available that contain the essential fatty acids, EPA and DHA, without the usual content of Vitamin A as retinol and Vitamin D. These specialised essential fats play a vital role at the end of pregnancy and in the first few months of life, in determining growth and development of the brain and eye. Again, supplements may be needed for those with a poor dietary intake.

CHAPTER 4

How to Improve Your Fertility

It takes two to make a pregnancy, and many of us manage it without any problems. However, approximately one in six couples will have some difficulty conceiving, which could be due to the woman's age, the man's sperm count or an assortment of other factors. About one in ten couples take more than a year to conceive, and one in twenty take more than two years. Even in the most fertile couples, the chance of becoming pregnant in each cycle is only 25 per cent, and some types of assisted conception approach this degree of success.

When the woman is aged under thirty-five, most couples need not rush into complex investigation: just follow those aspects of the advice given in this chapter that seem relevant. When the woman is aged thirty-five or more, or has significant disturbance of her menstrual cycle, then assessment after a year of regular intercourse is a reasonable guide.

Infertility is best viewed as a problem of the couple rather than just one of them. However, to understand the causes and treatments of infertility, it is easier to separate them into female and male. Many of the nutritional causes will overlap and self-help measures are as much for the couple as for the individual.

How Women Can Improve Their Fertility

Female fertility is determined by the health of the ovaries and their supply of eggs, the health of the fallopian tubes and uterus, the normal production of the hormones relating to reproduction by the pituitary gland at the base of the brain, and the ovaries themselves. Illness or problems with any of these will reduce the chances of fertility.

By the time a woman is born all the eggs that her ovaries will contain have already been produced! Several million eggs are in place initially, but only about 400 of them will reach maturity. The supply is influenced by smoking even before birth. The daughters of women who smoke in pregnancy have fewer eggs, may reach the menopause earlier and may have more difficulty conceiving compared to the offspring of non-smokers. Eggs, like sperm, are very sensitive to environmental factors.

The monthly release of an egg from the ovary is known as ovulation and occurs at approximately mid-cycle with menstruation, the monthly period, coming fourteen days later. Ovulation does not always occur with every cycle. It usually occurs during regular cycles of twenty-five to thirty-five days' duration, especially in women below the age of forty. This becomes much less certain, and therefore sub-fertility is more likely, in women with a very irregular cycle or who are over forty at the time of trying to conceive.

The egg which has been released from the ovary is picked up by the finger-shaped projections at the end of the fallopian tubes and then passes along toward the womb. Fertilisation actually takes place in the fallopian tube where the embryo, or recently fertilised egg, stays for several days, rapidly growing from one single cell into eight cells before passing on into the womb. Here it is implanted in the lining of the womb, or endometrium, by now about one week after ovulation.

The embryo produces a unique hormone, HCG – human

51

chorionic gonadotrophin – which passes via the bloodstream to the ovary, and stimulates it to continue its production of the female sex hormone, progesterone. In a non-fertile cycle the fall in the level of progesterone leads to the shedding of the lining of the womb – your monthly period. This obviously does not happen when fertilisation takes place. A missed period is often the first sign of pregnancy which can be confirmed by blood or urine tests that detect the presence of HCG.

In order for fertilisation to take place the fallopian tubes must be healthy, and not scarred by previous infection which would prevent the upward passage of sperm and the downward passage of the egg and embryo. Hormonal problems that cause the lining of the womb to be unreceptive to implantation can be another factor in infertility.

CAUSES OF FEMALE INFERTILITY
Investigations into female infertility look at many different possible causes.

Failure of Ovulation
This can be due to hormonal problems including an early menopause, an under- or over-active thyroid gland, disturbance of the pituitary gland (especially an excess of the hormone prolactin), and to excessive exercise, nutritional deficiencies and any chronic illness, especially if there is weight loss. Stress is a powerful factor in preventing ovulation.

The simplest guide to whether or not an egg is being produced each month is the regularity of the menstrual cycle which should be between twenty-five and thirty-five days. Regularity of ovulation can be checked by measuring the blood level of the female sex hormone progesterone seven days before the next period is due. Usually this is day 21 of a 28-day cycle, but will be day 28 in a 35-day cycle.

A rise in early morning body temperature of 0.5°C should

also be observed in the few days after ovulation, but this is less reliable than measuring the progesterone level. Often the day 21 progesterone level is checked in two or three cycles in couples with fertility problems, especially if there is some uncertainty about ovulation.

Most hormonal abnormalities are detected by blood tests. One of the commonest to be measured is prolactin which comes from the pituitary. An excessive amount in the blood inhibits ovulation. Often the first clues that this is the case are the presence of a milky white discharge from the nipples, known as galactorrhoea, and infrequent periods. However, only one-quarter of those with galactorrhoea will have a high prolactin level, and this then requires further investigation. High prolactin levels can be caused by stress, drugs (see page 57), an underactive thyroid, and pituitary problems.

Changing your diet can affect ovulation. Even following a 1,000 calorie weight-loss diet for six weeks may suppress normal ovulation. The World Health Organisation survey of infertility found that recent weight loss or gain was a mild risk for infertility.

Case History

EXERCISE AND INFERTILITY
Linda was a physical education teacher who was a keen long-distance runner. Her periods had stopped nine years earlier when she was nineteen and doing a lot of exercise. She then took the oral contraceptive pill for several years, and on stopping the pill her periods did not return for two years and then only after she received some hormonal treatment. Investigations by her gynaecologist showed only that she was not ovulating, and she was therefore given further hormonal treatment.

Nutritional tests revealed a very low level of magnesium in the red blood cells, as well as low zinc and essential fatty acid levels. She improved her diet, reduced the amount of running she was doing, and took supplements of magnesium, zinc, multi-vitamins and evening primrose oil. After these changes she was then treated with GIFT (gamete intrafallopian transfer, see page 60), and became pregnant, giving birth to a 2.72 kg (6 lb) baby girl the following year.

As in most cases it is impossible to determine the exact part played by each of these treatments. It makes sense to tackle the problem by looking at as many possible contributory factors and using a good degree of common sense in advising those with fertility problems.

Blockage of the Fallopian Tubes

This is another common cause of infertility which is very often due to past infection, most commonly by an organism called Chlamydia. It is usually acquired following sexual intercourse, and causes lower abdominal or pelvic pain, a vaginal discharge, painful periods and sometimes a fever. The acute illness is called pelvic inflammatory diseases (PID), and requires treatment with antibiotics. Often, however, the infection is silent. It and other related sexually acquired infections are more common in those who have had multiple partners and did not make use of barrier methods of contraception. The likelihood of pelvic inflammatory disease can be assessed:

★ from the history of sexually transmitted infection in either partner
★ from a vaginal examination, which might show evidence of active infection
★ from a blood test which can identify if there has been

past infection with chlamydia

To confirm the diagnosis a more detailed assessment by laparoscopy, examination of the pelvic organs with a telescopic instrument passed into the abdominal cavity, may be required. X-ray examination of the fallopian tubes will determine whether they are open or blocked. Residual or active infection requires antibiotic treatment. Blocked or damaged tubes can be corrected by surgery, but assisted fertilisation is often the simplest way to achieving pregnancy.

The reporting of infection with chlamydia more than doubled in the UK between 1976 and 1986, and damaged fallopian tubes is now the commonest cause of infertility in many developing countries because of the high prevalence of pelvic inflammatory disease.

Infection with other organisms, including gonorrhoea, are also important but less common causes of infertility due to fallopian tube blockage. Blocked or damaged tubes can be the result of past abdominal surgery – for appendicitis or almost any abdominal operation involving the ovaries or womb – especially if infection, such as peritonitis, was also present.

Endometriosis
In this condition, cells from the lining of the womb, the endometrium, can be situated in unusual sites such as around the ovaries or adjacent to the outer walls of the womb. Difficulty conceiving, very painful periods and abdominal distension are common problems. Diagnosis is often made after investigative surgery, a laparoscopy, to examine the pelvic organs. Unfortunately treatment is not very successful.

Polycystic Ovarian Disease
This condition is not uncommon and may be present in up to 20 per cent of the normal female population. It is character-ised by cysts on the ovaries and a shift in the balance of sex hormones resulting in:

★ irregular and infrequent periods
★ excessive hair growth
★ reduced fertility
★ and often, but not always, obesity

Associated with ovarian cysts is an underlying hormonal abnormality, of excess or increased sensitivity to the male sex hormone androgen, and a failure to ovulate regularly. The condition is diagnosed by blood tests and an ultra-sound scan which examines the ovaries. Losing weight if you are overweight, hormonal treatments and sometimes an operation to remove part of the affected ovary – a wedge resection – are the treatments used, and can promote fertility.

Contraception
This has only a small effect on subsequent fertility. Users of the oral contraceptive pill may experience a delay of a few months before they re-establish a normal menstrual cycle. This is not true infertility, but *delayed* fertility, as in the end they catch up with non-pill users in the rate at which they conceive. Users of intra-uterine devices have an increased risk of pelvic inflammatory disease, tubal damage and sub-sequent infertility, but this effect is slight.

Abortion
A history of abortion does not seem to reduce the future chance of conceiving according to recent research.

Medical Drugs
Many drugs can interfere with a woman's fertility. This is almost always reversible and can follow use of:

★ anti-cancer agents
★ hormone preparations as may be used to treat period pains or premenstrual problems
★ drugs used in the treatment of schizophrenia and depression
★ drugs metoclopramide and domperidone used in the treatment of nausea
★ and the drugs reserpine and methyldopa used in the treatment of high blood pressure, all of which can increase the level of the pituitary hormone prolactin

Medical Conditions
Diabetes and thyroid disease can cause infertility in women, but only if they are not well controlled.

Case History

Hilary was a 32-year-old shop manageress, who had been trying to become pregnant for the last four years. Infertility investigations had revealed no obvious defect in her or her husband, and she was about to embark upon a course of GIFT (gamete intrafallopian transfer). She just wanted to make sure that everything on the dietary side was fine.

Indeed it was. She was a non-smoker and non-drinker, and was eating an excellent diet with a good intake of protein, fruit and vegetables. Blood tests had shown good levels of iron, zinc and magnesium.

Examination, however, revealed a resting pulse rate of 128/minute, and a slightly enlarged thyroid. Tests confirmed that she was indeed thyrotoxic, and it was possible that this was contributing to her infertility problems. Her over-active thyroid was then controlled by drugs, and later she had an operation to remove part of the thyroid. Because of this and work changes she decided to defer starting a family.

An under- or over-active thyroid gland can be an occasional cause of infertility. Usually an over-active thyroid gland presents with symptoms of fatigue, tremor, heat intolerance, weight loss, sweating and palpitations, but she had none of these symptoms, though they undoubtedly would have followed were she not treated.

Social Poisons

Many, though not all, studies show slightly reduced fertility rates in those women who drink or smoke. Coffee consumption has also been studied, and there is a possible slight adverse effect on fertility. The same may be true of the consumption of soft drinks that have a high sugar content and contain colourings and additives. There are many other possible explanations including the associated dietary habits of those who smoke, drink alcohol or consume large amounts of coffee and soft drinks.

Recreational drugs including marijuana may reduce the chances of fertility. More importantly they can have a devastating effect on pregnancy outcome.

Environmental Chemicals

Studies that have looked at women's exposure to chemicals, especially in the work-place, have reported reduced fertility rates in association with textile and leather dyes, lead, mercury, benzene, petroleum and related chemicals, and possibly other chemicals used in the plastics industry. Female dental assistants have been reported as having delayed conception, possibly due to their exposure to the anaesthetic gas, nitrous oxide.

Nutritional Deficiencies

It is widely accepted in developing countries that a significant degree of malnutrition which results in severe weight loss is likely to stop a woman menstruating and could result in her being infertile. Surprisingly, there has been no concerted attempt to determine if *mild* nutritional deficiencies contribute to infertility in women from developed countries. Several small reports have documented the association of deficiencies of iron (without anaemia), Vitamin B12 and Vitamin B3 being associated with reduced fertility.

Other Causes

Rarely, structural abnormalities of the uterus or vagina may be a barrier to fertility, or prevent successful implantation of the fertilised ovum. Some women fail to menstruate at all because of genetic problems, but this is also very rare.

A few women produce antibodies to sperm or even have allergic reactions to it! Treatment with assisted conception can get round this problem.

Despite careful assessment of both partners, no cause for infertility is found in some 20 per cent of couples. Usually this diagnosis is made after laparoscopic examination of the woman, sperm counts and post-coital sperm examination in the man. Fortunately there is a high spontaneous pregnancy rate in those couples in this category. If spontaneous pregnancy has not occurred within three years, then some form of treatment is deemed appropriate.

TREATMENT OF FEMALE INFERTILITY

The treatment very much depends upon the cause. I outline the main types of treatment below, but in addition to the efforts of the gynaecologist there is quite a lot you can do to help yourself.

Failure of Ovulation

This is tackled in two main ways: by correcting any underlying hormonal abnormality, or by inducing ovulation through short courses of agents that encourage the ovary to release an egg.

These measures might be aided by attention to diet and lifestyle which we will come to shortly. Certain nutrients seem to play a crucial part in the way our ovaries respond to pituitary hormones (magnesium and possibly the essential fatty acids), and in influencing female sex hormone metabolism in general (Vitamin B, essential fatty acids and possibly magnesium and zinc). Severe deficiencies of these nutrients are rare except in women with very poor diets, or who are seriously ill or alcoholic. However there is now substantial evidence that mild undetected deficiencies are quite common, and they may have a modest effect upon the regularity of your menstrual cycle and ovulation.

Tubal Disease

Blockage or damage to the fallopian tubes can be treated in one of two ways: by surgery to repair the damaged tube(s), or by assisted conception.

Tubal repair surgery is surprisingly not very effective, as it is difficult to repair damage to the delicate tube lining, but it is useful for reversal of sterilisation procedures. Newer specialised techniques – trying to remove scar tissue from inside the fallopian tube by passing an ultrafine tube via the uterus – may be more successful.

Many couples in whom tubal disease is the main barrier to fertility will be best to opt for in-vitro fertilisation (test-tube fertilisation), using the partner's sperm and transfer of the fertilised egg to a receptive uterus.

Assisted Reproduction Techniques

This is very often the method of choice for women with tubal disease, unexplained infertility of more than three years' duration, and those with ovulation problems that have not responded to more simple measures. It can also help where the male partner has very few sperm or when the woman has no eggs and is willing to use donated eggs.

These techniques involve collection of a woman's eggs, often after treatment with hormonal agents, collection of sperm and their careful preparation. Then there is either in-vitro fertilisation (IVF or test-tube fertilisation) with placement of the embryo in the womb, or placement of both the prepared eggs and sperm in the fallopian tubes (gamete intrafallopian transfer or GIFT). In some circumstances it may be appropriate to use donor eggs from (usually) younger women together with the partner's sperm.

The disadvantages of these techniques are that they are highly specialised, stressful, costly (usually a few thousand pounds per attempt), and not without some health risk. Success rates are up to 25 per cent per cycle in selected cases. Many couples will need to undertake three or four attempts in order to succeed. Miscarriage rates are also increased, and no couple should embark upon this course without a very full understanding of the risks and possible outcomes, including multiple births.

How Men Can Improve Their Fertility

Sperm are produced in the testes by specialised cells, and slowly mature over four months. During orgasm they are ejected from the part of the testis called the seminiferous tubules, mix with fluid from the prostate gland and other tissues, and are released into the outside world. Millions are produced, even though only one is required to fertilise an egg. The number and quality of sperm as well as the health of the prostate gland are all important in deciding how fertile any one male is.

Sperm production takes place most efficiently at a temperature of 33°C, and thus the testicles are *outside* the body, which has a temperature of 37°C. Raising the temperature of the testes reduces the sperm count! A normal ejaculate should:

★ be greater than 2 ml (or millilitres)
★ contain at least 20 million sperm per ml
★ have 30 per cent or more with a normal shape
★ have 50 per cent actively mobile

As you can see, it is quite normal for some 50 per cent of sperm to be 'duds'. For sperm to be produced, a diet adequate in calories and protein is essential. The testicles have very high contents of zinc and Vitamin B, which seem to be important in sperm production.

Assessment of male infertility requires asking many questions about diet and lifestyle, a physical examination and an examination of a sample of sperm. Quite often a sperm sample can be collected by using a post-coital test: a sample is taken from the women's cervix some twelve hours after the couple have had intercourse. This tests not only sperm quantity and quality, but also how it responds to the partner's cervical mucus.

CAUSES OF MALE INFERTILITY
Investigations into male infertility look at many possible causes.

Absent or Deformed Testicles
Absent, small or enlarged testes can all be factors in male infertility. It is rare for testes to be absent, however. More usually they may have failed to descend from their original position high up in the scrotum or lower part of the abdomen. New-born and infant boys are routinely checked

to make sure the testes are descended. Small testes may be due to past injury, illness or sometimes developmental problems. Enlargement is most commonly due to a varicocele – enlargement of the veins around the testis – and this is present in 10 per cent of the normal population. This can raise the temperature of the testes, and contribute to a poor sperm count. Surgical treatment is often necessary.

Blockage of the Vas Deferens

Blockage of the duct leading from the testicles to the base of the bladder will result in a very low number or no sperm in the ejaculate. Previous vasectomy is an obvious cause, and can be reversed by surgery. Sometimes the sperm-carrying ducts are distorted as they reach the area of the prostate gland. Consequently some or all of the ejaculate does not reach the outside world directly, but passes into the bladder. Sperm are detected in the urine that is passed after inter-course. This commonly happens after surgery on the prostate gland.

Excessive Heat and the Testicles

Occupations that involve exposure to considerable heat can be associated with a reduced sperm count. This includes steel workers and bakers. Severe obesity and tight under-wear and trousers may play a part too.

Damage to the Testicles

Many factors actually damage the chromosomal material in the sperm itself, or reduce the amount or motility of the sperm. These include:

★ infection, especially sexually transmitted disease like chlamydia or non-specific urethritis (NSU)
★ infection with mumps during adolescence or early adult life

★ drugs as used for cancer and colitis or Crohn's disease
★ radiation treatment
★ exposure to environmental pollutants – lead, cadmium, mercury, pesticides, herbicides and other chemicals that have effects similar to the female sex hormone, oestrogen
★ cancer of the testicle

Chronic Illnesses
Diabetes, cystic fibrosis, chronic disease of the nervous system, any chronic infection or unexplained fever, an underactive thyroid gland, disease of the pituitary gland and kidney disease can all affect sperm count. Sperm counts also fall in men who are paralysed by a spinal injury.

Social Poisons
Alcohol and cigarette smoking are the most important, but marijuana and other recreational drugs can be factors too.

Lack of Essential Nutrients
Some nutrients seem to be particularly important to sperm production, and these include zinc, Vitamins B and C. One experiment in healthy volunteers of mild zinc deficiency showed a dramatic reduction in sperm quantity and quality, and testosterone (male sex hormone) production, which took nearly a year to fully correct.

Stress
Stress might also be a factor in reducing men's sperm count.

FALLING SPERM COUNT IN THE MODERN WORLD
A group of Danish doctors published an important review in 1992 of the fall in sperm count that seems to have taken place over the last fifty years. Looking at sixty-one papers detailing the results in nearly 15,000 men, there appears to have been a 40 per cent decline in sperm concentration and

a 20 per cent decline in seminal volume over this time. Combined with the known increase in testicular cancer and developmental abnormalities of the genitals in new-born boys, this strongly suggests an environmental cause, probably due to pollution.

Smoking, alcohol and lack of some essential nutrients may also be factors. The escalating use of the oral contraceptive pill and hormone replacement therapy, traces of which can find their way into the general environment, should give us all something to be concerned about. Increased use of plastics and related chemicals, the pesticide DDT and the chemical PCBs used as insulators for electrical cables prior to 1970, have also been suggested as factors, because of their mild oestrogen-like effects. Decline in reproductive capacity could be interpreted as an indication that the planet is becoming too crowded, and is Mother Nature's answer to the problem.

TREATMENT OF MALE INFERTILITY
This does of course depend upon the cause but unfortunately most of the treatments tried are not very successful. Self-help measures may be more effective at improving sperm count and function than are drug therapies.

Drugs
A wide variety of drugs and hormonal treatments, including steroids, have all been tried with either no benefit or uncertain benefit being recorded. Steroids can be useful in those men whose infertility is due to antibodies that attack their own sperm. Hormonal treatments are only helpful for the small percentage of men with true hormone deficiency.

Surgery
This is useful if blockage of the ducts from the testicles is causing a low sperm count. Enlargement of the veins of the testicles, a varicocele, can be treated by surgery if there is a

low sperm count, when infertility has been present for two or more years, and if there is no associated hormonal disturbance.

Antibiotics
These are necessary to treat any infection of the testicles or prostate gland. Treatment for several months may be required.

Assisted Reproduction Techniques (ART)
Modern techniques that bring together the sperm and egg, often outside the body (test-tube fertilisation or in-vitro fertilisation, IVF), are often the best hope for many couples where a low sperm count is the main barrier to conception. Such techniques involve collection of the partner's sperm, treatment with agents that improve its function, bringing together the sperm and egg – sometimes by actually injecting healthy sperm into the egg – and return of the fertilised egg into the womb. In this way pregnancy can be achieved when there is a very low sperm count.

If there is no sperm, then donor sperm will have to be used, and the donor can be chosen to have similar physical characteristics to those of the male partner.

SIMPLE SELF-HELP MEASURES

Whilst none of what follows may be as important as the hormonal and surgical techniques that have revolutionised female infertility treatment in particular, they all have their importance. It seems foolish not to take simple common-sense measures to improve health before embarking upon costly assisted reproduction techniques. Remember that most of the advice that follows will take three to six months before it has a detectable effect upon body chemistry and therefore a subsequent influence upon your reproductive ability.

BOTH

★ Cut down on alcohol and cigarettes – ideally stop. Cigarette smoking in women is associated with reduced fertility and means a lower success rate in those undergoing assisted reproduction techniques.

★ Eat a healthy diet with plenty of fresh fruit and vegetables. Their high content of Vitamins A, C and E act as antioxidants that help limit the adverse effects of many environmental pollutants. Ensure a good intake of protein-rich foods of either animal or vegetable origin: these are particularly important for men as they are good sources of zinc, which seems to play such a crucial role in sperm production and function.

★ If you are very overweight then lose weight, and if underweight try to gain weight, but always by eating healthy nutritious foods. Rapid weight change, gain or loss, is usually undesirable, in women especially.

★ If you are on long-term drug therapy ask your doctor or specialist to review your need for medication. The goal is the minimum effective dose for a drug or drugs, with the least risk of side-effects. In men, drug therapy for mental problems or Crohn's disease could be reducing sperm count.

★ If you have any chronic illness that is not being adequately treated at present, then check with your doctor.

★ Limit exposure to environmental chemicals. Take especial care if your work involves handling heavy metals, pesticides or industrial chemicals.

WOMEN

★ Limit consumption of tea and coffee to a total of four cups per day. More might have a small adverse effect on the chance of conceiving.

★ Do not consume more than three cans of soft drink, low calorie or normal type, per week. This is about 1 litre (1¾ pints) in volume.

★ Consider taking nutritional supplements, depending upon your health circumstances. Expert advice is often desirable and if you are receiving infertility treatment then you should always check with your specialist about these before commencing.

Iron may be needed by those who:

★ have heavy periods
★ are poorly fed, such as vegetarians who are also tea drinkers
★ have symptoms of iron deficiency, e.g. recurrent mouth ulcers or a sore tongue
★ have flattened or up-turned nails
★ have poor hair growth

Folic acid should be taken by all women who are trying to or who might conceive. The dose is 400 mcg per day.

Vitamin B Complex could be needed by those who:

★ eat poorly
★ consume more than an average of two units of alcohol daily
★ suffer from significant anxiety or depression
★ have any illness that has caused recent weight loss
★ have recurrent mouth ulcers or a sore tongue

Vitamin B12 may be needed by vegans. All women wishing to become pregnant should be taking folic acid, and it is a wise precaution that all vegans should also take a Vitamin B12 supplement. A mild deficiency of Vitamin B12 could be made worse by taking extra folic acid, resulting in damage to the nervous system and numbness in the hands or feet. An appropriate dose of Vitamin B12 is 5 mcg per day.

Magnesium might be helpful for those who are deficient, and have trouble ovulating regularly. Early symptoms that could indicate a lack of this essential mineral are:

★ premenstrual syndrome – physical or mental symptoms
★ muscle pains or cramps
★ fatigue

An appropriate dose is 300 mcg per day. Once pregnant, your need for these supplements may well change. Again check with your GP or specialist.

MEN

★ Avoid use of jockey-style underwear and underwear made from synthetic materials. Cotton boxer shorts will help keep the testicles at the right temperature.
★ If your sperm count is low, then rather than 'saving it all up for one good go' it would seem better to have more frequent intercourse, especially around mid-cycle. The optimum frequency of intercourse to maintain a good sperm count is two or three times a week. Recent research suggests that, in men with low counts, second ejaculates may contain more rather than less sperm than the first. So go to bed earlier and leave the dishes until the morning!
★ Do not have excessively hot baths or showers. Limit the time you spend in a sauna. Avoid exposure to excessively hot environments, at work for instance.
★ Take nutritional supplements of Vitamin C (about 500 mg), multi-vitamins and zinc (up to 30 mg) per day. These can all help improve sperm count, especially if you have low levels of Vitamin C. These moderate doses can be safely taken in the long term, but the positive effects are likely to take three or six months at least to be felt. Supplements of other nutrients may be needed if you

69

have deficiencies or other health problems.

Remember that all of these factors are likely to take some time to show results. Whilst getting yourselves into better condition, you will both need a little patience. If you haven't managed to conceive after two years of regular sexual intercourse you will need to see your doctor with a view to organising some specialist investigations. Most doctors do not initiate any treatment until after three years though this can be less in older couples.

CHAPTER 5

The Truth about Social Poisons

Some of our social vices, the things we so often enjoy, are bad for us, especially during our reproductive years. Alcohol, even in relatively moderate quantities, can cause life-long damage to your baby. Cigarette smoking has a direct effect on the size of your baby and its long-term health prospects. Caffeine, which is found in coffee, tea, cola-based drinks and chocolate, has been associated with spontaneous abortion and chromosomal abnormalities.

If you indulge in one or more of these on a regular basis you will need to take stock, ideally before you conceive. Consider the facts relating to each substance, and then assess whether you feel it would be wise to suffer a period of withdrawal and search out some alternatives.

ALCOHOL

In 1981 the Surgeon General of the United States stated that 'pregnant women, and those planning a pregnancy, should abstain from the use of alcohol'. This opinion was endorsed by the Royal College of Psychiatrists in 1982, and the Royal College of Physicians in 1987. The fact is that drinking alcohol during the preconceptual phase, or whilst you are pregnant, can cause serious physical and mental damage to your baby.

71

This may well come as a shock to you, as under normal circumstances many of us drink a few glasses of our favourite tipple each day without thinking for a moment that we are *over*-indulging.

The evidence that alcohol can damage the unborn child is not new. In 1973 a group of researchers described the many physical and mental developmental features seen in babies who had chronic alcoholic mothers, and coined the term Foetal Alcohol Syndrome. These include:

★ growth retardation
★ developmental deformities of the head and face
★ brain damage, resulting in mental handicap and possible spasticity
★ deformities of the heart
★ deformities of the skeleton

Whilst you might justifiably say that you are not an alcoholic, some of these defects have been found in babies born to women who were drinking much smaller amounts of alcohol on a regular basis. Although the effects of drinking moderate amounts of alcohol during pregnancy are controversial, most experts agree that it is best to err on the side of caution, and to abstain completely during this phase of your life.

Survey of 448 Mothers
ALCOHOL CONSUMPTION BEFORE THE LAST
PREGNANCY

25% of the women reduced their alcohol consumption in preparation
34.6% stopped alcohol altogether
14% did not change their drinking habits

23% were not drinkers
3 women drank *more* alcohol
10 women did not reply to the question

Women metabolise alcohol more slowly than men, probably because they usually have more spare fat, and it is the fatty tissue that absorbs the alcohol and releases it slowly into the system. It is then transported to the liver and broken down. The horrifying fact is that the baby receives alcohol *before* it is broken down by the mother. It receives it *neat*. Its immature liver, which doesn't start forming until some four weeks after conception, cannot possibly deal with the alcohol, and so damage occurs.

Survey of 448 Mothers
ALCOHOL CONSUMPTION DURING LAST PREGNANCY

Units per week	Number of women
7–10	3
5–6	9
3–4	23
1–2	79
0	330
No reply	4

There were 114 alcohol drinkers in our survey, which showed that women who drank as well as smoked had smaller babies.

As many women are unaware that they have conceived at this stage, it is likely that many would have consumed far too much alcohol during the preceding four months, which would put their unborn babies at risk. Knowing the risks attached to alcohol consumption is vital before you plan a pregnancy, which endorses the importance of a sound preconceptual programme as opposed to an unplanned pregnancy.

Case History

Heather was a 41-year-old whose first child, a daughter, was now five years old. Since then she had had four miscarriages at ten to eleven weeks, and this was almost certainly related to her drinking 1 litre (1¾ pints) of cheap wine every day!

She wanted to know what she could do to help her have another child. The advice was obvious, and was accompanied by recommendations to improve her diet and take some strong supplements of Vitamin B (including folic acid), zinc and magnesium, as investigations had shown marked deficiencies of these nutrients.

She was willing to do this but not to reduce her alcohol consumption. Over a few months she felt much better in herself: her depression lifted, premenstrual mood changes were less, and some mild eczema cleared. Eventually she cut down her drinking and then stopped altogether for a brief while.

She began drinking heavily again, consuming ten units daily, and a month later fell pregnant. Fortunately she was still taking her nutritional supplements and by the fifth week had managed to stop drinking again. At the twelfth week of pregnancy she experienced some slight bleeding but the pregnancy continued successfully, and she even developed an aversion to alcohol. She continued with her supplements to which some iron was added because of anaemia.

After forty-two weeks she gave birth to the healthy (3 kg, 7 lb) boy that she and her husband had wanted so much. She managed to breast-feed for several months, and during this time took multi-vitamins, calcium and evening primrose oil.

Alcohol consumption at ten units a day is associated with a greatly increased chance of miscarriage, and poor growth and developmental problems in a successful pregnancy (that appear to have been avoided in this instance).

SMOKING

Despite all the health-education campaigns that have been and gone, it is estimated that one in three women are still smoking at the time they discover they are pregnant. Repeated research shows that smoking causes:

★ spontaneous miscarriage
★ a malfunctioning placenta
★ congenital abnormalities
★ low birth weight
★ still-birth
★ increased illness like asthma and glue ear in young children
★ lower intelligence

It is also thought that up to 25 per cent of cot deaths are associated with smoking.

It is estimated that 28 per cent of mothers in the UK smoke during pregnancy, and in the USA 26 per cent continue to smoke through their pregnancy.

Survey of 448 Mothers
CIGARETTE SMOKING BEFORE PREGNANCY

---

156 women in our group were smokers
12.5% of women in our sample stopped smoking before their last pregnancy
10.7% did not change their smoking habits
10.3% cut down on their consumption
6 women increased their smoking before getting pregnant.
62.5% were non-smokers

Our survey also showed that smokers had smaller babies than non-smokers.

Women who smoke during pregnancy double their risk of having low birth-weight babies, often as much as 200 g (7 oz) lighter than the babies of non-smokers.

Women who smoke during pregnancy double their chances of having delinquent children, which is thought to be a result of subtle brain damage during the developmental stages.

St George's Hospital birth weight study found that the diet of smokers was less nutritious than that of non-smokers during pregnancy. When smokers improved their diets by consuming more zinc, thiamin (Vitamin B1) and riboflavin (Vitamin B2) at thirty-six weeks, it had a positive effect on the birth weights of their babies. There is some evidence that the absorption of zinc, which is necessary for growth and development, is impaired by smoking.

THE SMOKE YOU INHALE
When you draw on a cigarette, the nicotine that you absorb causes important arteries to go into spasm, including those

in the placenta and the uterus. The result is that the baby receives a reduced supply of blood, oxygen and nutrients. This is probably the reason why smokers have smaller babies.

There are some 4,000 chemicals in tobacco smoke, only one of which is nicotine! Carbon monoxide, generated from cigarette and cigar smoking, also displaces oxygen in red blood cells, which is another reason why the baby receives an inferior supply.

By breathing in the carbon monoxide from 'second-hand' smoke – passive smoking – you will also be restricting the oxygen that reaches your baby. Research shows quite clearly that babies are more than twice as likely to have deformed faces if their fathers were heavy smokers.

So the message is don't smoke and don't spend much time in a smoky environment. If both you and your partner smoke, discuss the possibility of giving up together, preferably before you conceive. If only one of you smokes, then the non-smoker will have to be the supporter during the difficult days of withdrawal symptoms.

Survey of 448 Mothers
CIGARETTE CONSUMPTION DURING LAST PREGNANCY

Number of Women	Cigarettes per Day
3	25–30
7	29–16
8	11–15
29	10
14	5–9
9	1–4
372	None
6	No reply

There were 70 smokers in our sample. Our survey showed that women who smoked during their pregnancy had smaller babies than those who did not.

GIVING UP

No-one ever said that giving up smoking was easy. It requires both will-power and determination, as you are likely to go through withdrawal symptoms which are similar to those experienced by drug addicts and alcoholics. You have probably never had better motivation than a planned baby, so in that sense it may be easier. Also, if you are one of the lucky ones, you will find that you have little desire to smoke during pregnancy, and possibly even find the smell of tobacco repulsive, as your sense of smell is heightened. Making the decision to stop smoking is the first step, often followed by a sense of bewilderment about how to go about it, and self-doubt about whether you will be able to achieve it. Your stop-smoking plan should run rather like this.

★ Choose a day on which to give up, and write down the date.
★ On the day before, smoke as many cigarettes as you can until you feel sick. Make sure you stub them out in the same dirty ashtray.
★ Go to the library and get a book that contains pictures of the consequences of smoking.
★ On the morning of your chosen day, pour yourself a glass of freshly squeezed orange juice and sit and write out all the reasons for your decision to give up smoking.
★ Pin your list of reasons up on the wall so that you can read it at weak moments.
★ Put your cigarettes away in a drawer, and tell yourself you can have one whenever you want one.
★ When you crave for a cigarette, tell yourself you can have

one but first consider the reasons why you decided to quit. Make a new decision not to light up.

★ Go shopping and stock up with some of your favourite wholesome food, including some fruit and some raw vegetables and dips.

★ Tell your close friends and family that you are giving up smoking.

★ Take a good multi-vitamin and mineral pill each day, if you cannot improve your diet.

★ Try to avoid situations that are likely to make you feel like lighting up. For example, drink fruit juice instead of alcohol.

★ If possible, go away for a few days to help you break your daily routine.

★ Chew some sugar-free gum rather than sweets or chocolate.

★ Put the handle of your toothbrush in your mouth whenever you miss your hand-to-mouth habit.

★ Each time you feel you need a cigarette, stop, relax and breathe deeply, so that you get a good supply of oxygen into your lungs.

★ Join a gym, and make sure you exercise regularly.

★ Don't spend evenings alone: arrange to go to the cinema, bowling or out for a walk.

★ If you feel edgy in the evenings, have a few early nights.

★ Keep a progress chart, ticking each day you have remained a non-smoker.

★ Save your cigarette money in a jar, and spend it on treats for yourself.

★ Practise some formal kind of relaxation like yoga or meditation.

★ Get your partner to give you a massage when you feel a bit ratty or tense.

★ Look through baby books at pictures of lovely healthy babies and try to imagine what your healthy baby will look like with a good oxygen supply and optimum growth.

It is never too late to give up smoking. Whenever you take the plunge you will be improving the health of your loved ones as well as yourself. If you find it difficult to quit, contact one of the organisations listed on page 281.

Caffeine

Caffeine, which is a stimulant, crosses from the mother through the placenta to the unborn baby, so it is well worth while trying to cut down and stop coffee drinking before you become pregnant. Many women develop an aversion to coffee whilst they are pregnant, and although no scientific basis for this has been discovered it is likely that it is Mother Nature's way of helping us to protect our unborn children.

Caffeine is found in high concentrations in coffee, particularly ground coffee, which contains approximately 150 mg per mug. A mug of instant coffee contains about 100 mg, and a mug of tea roughly 80–100 mg. Caffeine is also present in cola-based drinks, chocolate and some painkillers that are available over the counter. In larger doses, however, symptoms which may be mistaken for 'anxiety neurosis' may develop: these include insomnia, irritability, anxiety, headaches, tremors, nausea and diarrhoea. Under normal circumstances, if we are well, moderate doses of up to 300 mg caffeine can improve performance and elevate our mood. However, during pregnancy we become more sensitive to caffeine, which means that the effect of one cup of coffee during pregnancy is equivalent to two at any other time.

Coffee is the most widely used drug of our time, but, although there is no strong evidence linking consumption with developmental problems in pregnancy, the stimulant effect on the baby must be considered. Because caffeine is passed across the placenta, it follows that if we feel 'hyped-up', then the baby is likely to suffer the effects also. Breast-fed babies of mothers who consume lots of coffee do seem to become restless and wakeful.

Decaffeinated drinks contain many of other substances that can cause problems, so they are not a real solution in any quantity. There are, however, many coffee substitutes that are cereal based, which are worth a try. Barley Cup, dandelion coffee, Bambu and Caro can all be found in your local health-food shop, and are unlikely to produce any side-effects. Try to give up coffee *before* you become pregnant.

Survey of 448 Mothers
TEA AND COFFEE CONSUMPTION DURING PREGNANCY

11.4 per cent of our sample didn't drink either tea or coffee or didn't answer. Out of the tea and coffee drinkers, the average number of cups of tea per day was 3.1 and 1.5 cups of coffee.

Number of women	Tea cups/day
9	10–20
18	7–9
72	5–6
118	3–4
98	1–2
129	0
4	No reply

Number of women	Coffee cups/day
2	10–14
8	7–9

21	5–6
50	3–4
148	1–2
205	0
14	No reply

Women who drank more than 3 cups of coffee per day appeared to have slightly smaller babies, but this could be partly because many were also smokers.

STREET DRUGS

In an ideal world, women who are addicted to drugs should not have babies. Women using hard drugs like heroin, cocaine or crack pass on their addiction to the new-born baby. The baby often has to be weaned off the drug at birth, and suffer the painful withdrawal symptoms, which adults find difficult enough to deal with. The drugs often cause developmental problems, as well as behaviour disorders in childhood, and many children born to drug addicts are taken into care during the first ten years of their life.

COCAINE AND CRACK
Both cocaine and crack, the relatively recent, *purer* form of cocaine, have become increasingly popular in the last fifteen years. Unlike cocaine, crack is smoked, and this is absorbed more rapidly into the body. A study published in 1994, conducted in Amsterdam on a group of twenty-one mothers addicted to cocaine, and their twenty-three offspring, showed some very distressing results.

★ There were six premature babies.
★ Five babies had a small head circumference.

★ Two babies were small for their dates.
★ Three babies had congenital malformation.
★ One died shortly before birth.
★ One had congenital syphilis.
★ Four had permanent brain damage.
★ A further four had neurological damage, which might be permanent.
★ One died twenty-one days after birth.
★ At follow-up, four infants showed abnormal development.

HEROIN

Derived from the opium plant, heroin is another highly addictive drug that produces addicted babies that are also likely to be physically and mentally disadvantaged. Women who use heroin during pregnancy are three times more likely to miscarry or have a still-birth, and four times more likely to go into premature labour.

Studies have shown that babies born to heroin addicts were smaller, had slower growth and neurological development, were less intelligent, less socially competent, and had more behaviour disorders. The same problems were experienced by babies of women who were taking methadone, the replacement drug used during heroin withdrawals.

AMPHETAMINE

Addiction to amphetamines during pregnancy also has serious repercussions on new-born babies, but it does not stop there. A recent ten-year follow-up study was conducted in Holland. Sixty-five children who were born to amphetamine-addicted mothers were followed from birth.

★ 20 per cent of the children were put in foster homes at birth.
★ By the age of ten, 70 per cent were in foster homes.
★ At four years of age, 35 per cent showed aggressive behaviour.

★ At eight years of age, 23 per cent were still aggressive.
★ At ten, 12 per cent were in lower classes than their age.

Once again it seems that drug abuse during pregnancy has severe repercussions on the development of addicts' children.

MARIJUANA AND CANNABIS

Both of these widely used substances are products of the hemp plant, and are even legally available in some countries. The pro-marijuana lobby claim that it is as safe as smoking cigarettes or drinking alcohol. Seeing as neither cigarettes nor alcohol are being recommended during pregnancy, I am not about to suggest that you indulge in 'pot' smoking either.

The active ingredient in marijuana and cannabis is called tetrahydrocannabinol (THC), which is a steroid hormone related to oestrogen and progesterone. THC tends to accumulate in the ovaries and can severely upset the menstrual cycle, and can slow down the process of labour. These drugs have been shown to slow down the growth rate of developing babies, probably because of the increased intake of carbon monoxide in the smoke, and are even thought to be responsible for damage to the baby's chromosomes.

Surely no sane person could wish any of these curses on an innocent baby. If you use any drug, especially an addictive one, it is vital that you seek help and kick the habit before you attempt to conceive. Your doctor will be able to refer you to a specialist clinic. There are a few good books on overcoming addiction listed on page 275.

MEDICINES

This is an important aspect of health care before conception, as well as during pregnancy and breast-feeding. The prime functions of the placenta and breast are to pass nutrients from mother to baby in a high concentration, and many drugs are simply treated in the same way as nutrients. Thus what mother takes, baby will get too. Unfortunately, the baby's liver is not able to cope with the drug, and the sensitive growing cells may be unduly affected by even small doses that are well tolerated by the mother. This applies not only to drugs but to high-strength vitamin and mineral supplements and many herbal medicines. This is an area where there is no substitute for expert advice.

If you are on long-term therapy, no matter what it is, always check with your doctor first before becoming pregnant. Where possible, it is good practice to keep to a minimum the number and dosage of drugs that you take before conceiving. Where this is not possible, additional attention to diet and sometimes nutritional supplements are required to minimise the potential adverse effects of drugs upon the baby.

The following categories are worthy of special mention.

EPILEPTIC DRUGS
If taken during pregnancy these can affect the baby's immune system and development. Because many have an adverse effect on folic acid and Vitamin E, additional supplements of these nutrients should probably be taken by the majority of women prior to conception and certainly during the first three months, if not throughout the whole pregnancy.

ANTI-DEPRESSANTS
Specialist advice is required. Some of the side-effects of tricydic and anti-depressant drugs can be minimised by correcting any pre-existing mild deficiency of Vitamin B. Ensuring a healthy diet that is high in B vitamins may help. Again, the dosage should be reduced to a minimum and

whenever possible stopped for several months prior to conception.

ANTI-CANCER DRUGS
These are powerful drugs which interfere with cell growth. Many cause temporary sterility or greatly increase the risk of miscarriage. Take the advice of your specialist who will almost certainly advise contraception during treatment with anti-cancer drugs and probably to wait six months after they have ceased before trying to become pregnant.

ANTIBIOTICS
Tetracycline antibiotics – often used in the treatment of acne – will discolour and damage the baby's teeth if taken during pregnancy. Try trimethoprin and sulphonamide. Antibiotics often used for urinary tract infections interfere with the metabolism of folic acid and are unwise during the preconceptual phase and in early pregnancy. Metronidazole antibiotic used in the treatment of some vaginal and pelvic infections is not advisable until the seventh week of pregnancy. Other antibiotics, such as penicillin, are usually safer.

SEDATIVES
Sedative drugs such as diazepam are undesirable during pregnancy. They should be withdrawn several weeks before labour, otherwise the new-born infant may experience a withdrawal syndrome.

DRUGS FOR HIGH BLOOD PRESSURE
Some of these are safe during pregnancy, but again expert advice is usually required. Diuretics, which are often extremely safe in non-pregnant women, may alter placental blood supply.

STEROIDS

These drugs are often used in the treatment of allergies such as asthma and eczema, as well as severe forms of chronic arthritis. Again, the dosage should be reduced to a minimum, under expert guidance. Sudden reductions may be disastrous for the mother. Inhaled steroid sprays, if used in small doses, seem to be very safe. Again, if you require regular use of inhaled steroids for your asthma, reviewing the need for this by your doctor or specialist is a good idea.

PAINKILLERS

Many simple painkillers, including aspirin and paracetamol, appear to be relatively safe during the preconceptual period of pregnancy. However, if it is at all possible to do without them, or minimise the use of them, then this must be good policy. Eating a healthy diet and avoiding other toxins, including cigarettes and alcohol, will probably help to reduce the risk of adverse drug effects in pregnancy. The original animal experiments on thalidomide showed that in rats who were fed an adequate diet, thalidomide caused no congenital defects. When the laboratory diet was replaced with one deficient in Vitamins B or E, the all-too-familiar effects of thalidomide were rapidly apparent.

CHAPTER 6

Factfile on Miscarriage

Miscarriage is defined medically as the loss of any pregnancy before twenty weeks' gestation. There are many known causes and probably some unknown causes as to why women have miscarriages. The exact percentage of actual pregnancies that miscarry is not known precisely, although approximately 15 per cent of all recognised pregnancies miscarry. However, a pregnancy which miscarries within the first two weeks of conception is unlikely to be recognised as a miscarriage. A period may be a few days late and heavy, but otherwise the woman may not suspect that she actually conceived.

Survey of 448 Mothers
FREQUENCY OF MISCARRIAGES

---

103 women had one or more miscarriages (23%)
9 of these women had had three or more miscarriages (2%)
35 women had one or more terminations (8%)

A couple who are unfortunate enough to have a pregnancy end in miscarriage are probably likely to conceive again. Some women have recurrent miscarriages, three or more consecutive failed pregnancies before twenty weeks' gestation. In theory this should occur in less than half of 1 per cent of women but in effect occurs in approximately 1 per cent. Even so, over half the women who experience three miscarriages may still have a successful pregnancy despite their frustration and disappointment beforehand.

Case History

Vivienne was a 40-year-old chemist who had been married for fifteen years. During this time she had not used contraception, and had not fallen pregnant until just recently. She and her husband were delighted. However she was not in the best of health: generalised aches and pains and a feeling of malaise had troubled her for the last three years. Unfortunately the baby was still-born at thirty-nine weeks due to placental insufficiency. She conceived a second time but miscarried after three months.

At this time she was being investigated by another specialist for arthritis because now some of her joints had become swollen as well as painful. These tests revealed the presence of antibodies in her blood that attacked her own tissues. The one detected was called anti-cardiolipin antibody which is not uncommon in women with recurrent miscarriages, and was almost certainly the cause of her aches and pains. No treatment was required but she might be helped by taking a small amount of aspirin if she became pregnant. She was given some hormonal treatments to help her conceive.

89

THE CAUSES OF MISCARRIAGE

Miscarriage can be caused by many factors:

★ genetic problems – due to defects in chromosome or material from either partner
★ environmental factors, including smoking and drugs
★ hormonal abnormalities
★ pre-existing disease or medical conditions in the womb.

CHROMOSOME ABNORMALITIES

This is probably the main cause of sporadic or one-off miscarriages. It is Mother Nature's way of deciding not to continue with a pregnancy that might have resulted in a handicapped or significantly deformed child. The risk of miscarriage for this reason may be increased if there is a history of genetic illness in either partner's family or if the partners are related, e.g. cousins.

Increasing age of the mother is associated with an increase in miscarriage rate, possibly because of the greater likelihood of chromosomal damage to the eggs. Healthy diet and limiting exposure to environmental toxins and radiation in the mother from the time of conception to the time of reproduction might minimise the chance of genetic abnormalities occurring. Down's syndrome, a common genetic abnormality, is strongly related to increasing age of the mother because of the greater opportunity that this gives for spontaneous chromosomal abnormalities to develop in the egg prior to conception (see page 137).

SMOKING

Smoking is about the commonest environmental hazard associated with miscarriage. Smokers are approximately a quarter more likely to have a pregnancy end in miscarriage than non-smokers. Passive smoking might also raise the risk of miscarriage. The message is simple – stop smoking for three or four months before trying to conceive again. In our survey smoking was strongly related to the number of miscarriages: 28.6 per cent of smokers had miscarried once or more whereas only 21.4 per cent of non-smokers had. Overall, the rate of miscarriage in smokers was nearly twice that in non-smokers.

ALCOHOL AND DRUGS
Heavy alcohol consumption is certainly linked to a lower chance of successful outcome for pregnancy. Many illicit drugs carry a similar risk. Associated nutritional problems due to dietary neglect or the adverse effect of alcohol upon nutrition, are likely to be contributing factors.

NUTRITIONAL DEFICIENCIES
These might also be a factor in recurrent miscarriage. Malnutrition from a lack of calories and protein is usually obvious and during episodes of starvation that occurred during and after World War Two, increased rates of miscarriage were recorded.

Some other nutrients may be particularly important. In some women with recurrent miscarriage a relative lack of the chemicals required for the growth and development of blood vessels of the placenta was recorded. This chemical, prostacyclin, is derived from the important essential fatty acids found in seed oils e.g. sunflower oil. Adequate supply of zinc, Vitamin B, magnesium and other nutrients may also be necessary for the right biochemical environment for the early survival of the embryo.

HEAVY METALS
Lead and cadmium are two toxic minerals, increased amounts of which have been found in the tissues of still-born

babies. We are all exposed to these elements which have worked their way from industrial and other sources into our food and water supply. Cadmium in particular, present in cigarette smoke and lead, has of course come from petrol. The levels of lead are, however, falling significantly since the introduction of lead-free petrol. These metals are more toxic if the diet lacks essential nutrients, especially calcium, zinc and iron. A very poor intake of iron, calcium and zinc in the diet increases the risk of miscarriage.

PROBLEMS IN THE MOTHER'S ANATOMY
Miscarriage can be due to abnormalities of the genital tract, often a soft or weakened cervix, neck of the womb, that allows a late miscarriage to occur. Surgical treatment may be necessary prior to a subsequent conception, or the cervix may need stitching once pregnant.

HORMONAL IMBALANCES
Serious hormonal imbalances are more associated with infertility but might also result in miscarriage as well. Recent research has shown that increased levels of the pituitary hormone LH (luteinising hormone) close to conception and a low level of the ovarian hormone progesterone shortly after conception may reduce the chances of a successful outcome. These relatively minor hormonal imbalances in association with mild and usually silent ovarian cysts may be present in a high percentage of patients with recurrent miscarriages.

Obesity, poor diet and lack of essential nutrients that contribute to normal hormonal function might also be factors in disturbing the mother's delicate hormone chemistry which appears crucial to the survival of the pregnancy. Using hormonal preparations in early pregnancy is not a common practice as it is not considered to be very effective. Improving the mother's general health, including her nutritional state, is the best approach prior to the next pregnancy.

Disturbances in thyroid function can also increase the risk of miscarriage, but this is no greater than average when thyroid disease is treated.

POOR HEALTH

Conditions such as diabetes, high blood pressure and rare diseases that affect metabolism, may be associated with increased rates of miscarriage. Careful control of the medical condition prior to and after conception is essential.

Certain blood abnormalities associated with arthritis, such as back problems in women, are an important cause of recurrent miscarriage.

A condition called SLE – systemic lupus erythematosus – that causes arthritis, skin disorders and other problems in young women, is a known cause of recurrent miscarriage. The blood of such women and others, who may be identified only because they have recurrent miscarriages, may contain what are termed antiphospholipid antibodies. Sophisticated tests can now be performed to detect these, and this has become routine for many women who have experienced three consecutive miscarriages, for instance. Such blood abnormalities may lead to disturbance in the blood formation in the blood vessels in the placenta, and result in miscarriage or a still-birth later in the pregnancy. Specialist treatment prior to conception is necessary.

PREGNANCY SPACING

Miscarriages are slightly more likely to occur in pregnancies which follow within one year of a previous pregnancy. The spacing of two years allows time for the mother to improve her nutritional status.

INFECTION

It is well known that a variety of infections, including rubella (German measles) and Listeria, infection from 'live' soft cheeses, if contracted during early pregnancy can lead to miscarriage or congenital deformity. More recently, low-grade mild bacterial infection of the vagina has been linked to recurrency in miscarriage.

Some authorities recommend careful assessment of women with a history of miscarriage, especially if they have symptoms of vaginal infection, such as discharge, an offensive smell, vaginal irritation or urinary symptoms, including urinary frequency and pain. Antibiotic treatment by mouth or pessary is usually required to clear such infection prior to attempting any further pregnancy.

The most sinister bacterial cultures appear to be Gardnerella vaginalis and Mycoplasma hominis. Their presence, together with reduced numbers of the healthy Lactobacillus, is associated with a several-fold increased risk of miscarriage between sixteen and twenty-four weeks' gestation, as well as an increased risk of pre-term labour. These, and other related infections, may be present in approximately 10 per cent of women. They require treatment prior to conception or, if found during a pregnancy, prior to delivery.

WHAT CAN YOU DO ABOUT MISCARRIAGE

The first thing to do if you have just had one miscarriage is not to worry. Wait at least three months before trying to conceive again, and in this time make any necessary changes to your diet, modify your consumption of alcohol and/or cigarettes and, if you have an existing medical problem which is not being well managed, then make an appointment to see your doctor or specialist. There is no need to worry. Simply try to conceive again when your body feels ready.

If you need to use contraception whilst waiting, then it is best to use a barrier method for this purpose.

Specialist tests are not normally required for those with a one-off miscarriage.

For women with recurrent miscarriage, a test to look for new abnormalities – phospholipid antibodies and chromasomal abnormalities – is becoming routine. Hormonal investigation may also be required, depending upon the mother's menstrual history.

Chromosome and immune abnormalities are unlikely to be improved by attention to nutritional state. Mild hormonal abnormalities might respond to attention to the mother's diet as well as appropriate hormonal treatment.

Vaginal swabs can assess the possibility of infection. If you are at all concerned, go along to discuss the situation with your doctor. It is not all bad news by any means.

CHAPTER 7

Your Preconceptual Programme

You have probably gathered by now that both you and your partner need to be in tip-top condition before thinking about conceiving. There are a number of preparation steps that you should take in the six months prior to even thinking of starting a baby. Once you are both in peak condition your chances of conceiving quickly will be higher, so in the long run you will not have 'wasted' much time.

★ Follow the diet plan outlined on page 43 for at least four months, and get your partner to follow a similar diet, perhaps eating extra quantities if he is larger than you.
★ Take care to avoid all the foods and drinks which have been shown to impede the absorption of good nutrients or might harm your chances of a healthy baby, see pages 67–70.
★ Ideally both you and your partner should avoid drinking alcohol. At most, consume no more than three units per week.
★ You should spend at least four months in a smoke-free environment. That means that neither you nor your partner should be smoking, and you should avoid smoky atmospheres.
★ Take a multi-vitamin and mineral supplement that contains 400 mcg of folic acid and Vitamin B12, but not

Vitamin A (as retinol). Sanatogen Pronatal is a good example of a tailor-made pill, and is now available in all chemists and supermarkets.

★ If either you or your partner are concerned about your nutritional status, you could contact one of the organisations listed in the Women's Health section of the Appendix to arrange for appropriate blood tests.

★ If you suffer with fatigue, have pale skin and heavy periods, you should ask your doctor to check your serum ferritin levels, which will determine whether you have low iron stores.

★ Ask your doctor to check to see whether you are up to date with your rubella immunisation. It is important to be immune to German measles because it can cause so much irreversible damage to an unborn child if contracted in the first few weeks of pregnancy.

★ Your doctor will be happy to arrange for you to have a thorough check up to ensure that:
    * your blood pressure is in the normal range
    * you are free of diabetes
    * you have no pelvic problems
    * you have no vaginal or bladder infections
    * you are not an HIV carrier
    * you do not have any sexually transmitted disease

★ Take three or four good sessions of exercise per week, and try to get outdoors as often as possible, especially when it is sunny.

★ If you have been taking the contraceptive pill you will need to stop six months before you plan to conceive. The pill can interfere with essential vitamin and mineral levels.

★ If you have had an IUD fitted you will need to have it removed at least six months before you plan to conceive. The IUD can increase the risk of vaginal infection.

★ Use natural methods of contraception during your

97

preconceptual programme. Getting to know your body and learning to recognise when you are ovulating (see below) will help you in the long term to know when it is right to conceive.

★ Ideally you should not be taking any medication during pregnancy that is not absolutely necessary. If you are taking prescribed drugs, discuss the situation with your doctor to see whether there is any need for you to reduce your medication or to switch to an alternative prior to trying for a baby.

★ If either you or your partner use street drugs you will need to stop either with the support of each other if it's a social habit, or with the help of a clinic if you are addicted.

★ Avoid chemicals wherever possible for reasons that are more fully explained in Chapter Nine. You should:
  * use lead-free petrol
  * use ecologically safe cleaning creams at home
  * avoid using aerosols
  * avoid using any chemicals if you are a keen gardener or grow vegetables
  * avoid sitting for too long in front of a VDU on a regular basis
  * do not use copper or aluminium saucepans
  * only use the microwave for reheating or defrosting
  * keep away from busy main roads – if you live on one try to move
  * not spray pets with chemicals to prevent fleas
  * avoid paint which contains lead, and should not sleep in a freshly painted room
  * not use a sunbed whilst you are pregnant
  * use a hot water bottle to heat your bed rather than an electric blanket
  * sort out areas of stress in your personal or work life before you conceive

When both you and your partner have been following your preconceptual programme for at least four months, and preferably six, you will be ready to start thinking about conception.

Getting The Timing Right

A new egg is usually released by the ovary approximately fourteen days before your next period is due to start, and this process is known as ovulation. The first day of your cycle is the day your period begins. So for example if you have a 25-day cycle, you may ovulate on the eleventh day, whereas if you have a 34-day cycle, ovulation may not occur until the twentieth day of your cycle. For the majority of women who have a regular 28-day cycle, they can expect to ovulate around mid-cycle.

HOW TO IDENTIFY OVULATION TIME
Our bodies are terribly good at communicating about what is going on, the only problem is that we don't always know how to interpret the messages! There are several physical signs of ovulation, some of which are more obvious than others.

Mid-cycle Pain
Some women experience some pain or discomfort in their abdomen at the time of ovulation, which is a result of leakage of some of the fluid surrounding the egg as it is released into the fallopian tube. If you do experience this to some degree, and had previously regarded it as a nuisance, you will now come to realise that you are at a distinct advantage as you know precisely when the egg is being released.

Changing Mucus

It is quite normal to have a discharge from the vagina throughout your cycle. On non-fertile days the discharge is usually cloudy, sticky and thick, and designed to keep sperm out. As the process of ovulation begins the mucus changes dramatically, becoming 'wet', slippery, more transparent and stretchy, a bit like the consistency of egg white. If you are willing to test your mucus at different times of the cycle, you will find that during the fertile days it will stretch into an unbroken thread between your thumb and finger. Some women make more discharge than others, which makes the recognition process more obvious.

Temperature Change

Your body temperature drops slightly just before you ovulate, and then rises back to a higher level when the process of ovulation is complete. If you decide to keep a temperature chart you will need to obtain a special ovulation thermometer, called a basal thermometer, which is particularly sensitive, and measure your temperature every morning before rising, and certainly before eating or drinking. You may need to keep a temperature chart for several months before being certain of the pattern. It is easier to spot the rise in temperature after ovulation perhaps than to see the small drop that occurs prior to ovulation.

Ovulation Kit

If you want to see 'test-tube' evidence of ovulation, you could use one of the kits that are available over the counter at the chemist. At the onset of ovulation there is a surge of a hormone called luteinising hormone (LH) in your urine. The ovulation kits measure LH for five consecutive days or so towards mid-cycle. Usually ovulation follows between twelve and thirty-six hours after the LH surge. Once you have recorded a surge in LH you can make love, knowing that you are at the most fertile time of your cycle.

How long will it take to become pregnant?
Statistics show that some 80 per cent of couples manage to successfully conceive within the first year of trying. A lucky 38 per cent of non-smoking women fall pregnant during the first cycle that they try, compared to 28 per cent of women who smoke. Age plays a part too. Women in their twenties are likely to conceive more quickly than women who are in their mid to late thirties.

Unless you have been trying to conceive for more than a year, in which case you should probably have a chat with your doctor anyway, you are best advised to relax, let nature take its course and not get too mechanical about the act of conceiving. Continuing to enjoy a loving relationship without getting too neurotic about making a baby is in fact much more conducive to being successful, and will certainly make you feel happier.

Abstaining from intercourse for several days prior to ovulation is not now thought to be a wise move, as the volume of sperm may be affected by not making love regularly. Only making love once at the time of ovulation also will not necessarily be to your best advantage, as it seems that the sperm mobility from the second ejaculation is even better than the first.

DIET FOR PRECONCEPTION AND EARLY PREGNANCY

Sample Menus

Breakfast	Lunch	Dinner
DAY 1		
Jordans Muesli with chopped pear and almonds	Mackerel in tomato sauce	Lamb chops
Bio yoghurt and milk	Jacket potato	Carrots, cabbage and sweet-corn
Dandelion coffee	Mixed green salad	Fruit compote
	Pineapple juice	Hazelnut biscuits
	Fresh dates	Rooibosch tea
DAY 2		
Cornflakes with banana	Avocado with walnut oil and lemon dressing	Steamed salmon
Pecan nuts and raisins	Mung beans, alfalfa and tomato salad with Ryvita	New potatoes, peas, spinach
Bio yoghurt and milk		Grilled grapefruit with brown sugar topping
	Orange juice	Grapefruit juice with ginger ale
	Slice of melon	
DAY 3		
Scrambled eggs with tomatoes and mushrooms	Herring Roe on wholemeal toast with watercress and fennel salad	Duck with orange sauce
Wholemeal toast with orange marmalade	Satsumas	Brown rice with fried onions, parsnips and brussel sprouts
Rooibosch Eleven 'o'clock tea	Grapefruit juice	Mixed berry dessert with bio yoghurt
DAY 4		
Jordan's Oat Crunchy Cereal with grapes, walnuts and sesame seeds	Cauliflower cheese with jacket potato	Steak, home-made chips, peas and mixed salad
Bio yoghurt and milk	Fresh orange	Baked pears with Creme Fraiche
Decaffeinated coffee	Tomato juice	Banana and cinnamon tea
DAY 5		
2 hardboiled eggs	Sardines with wholemeal toast, watercress, red pepper and cucumber salad	Stir-fry broccoli and seaweed with almonds, egg and fried rice
Ryvita		
Orange marmalade	Glass of milk	Citrus fruit salad with cream
Dandelion coffee	Fresh strawberries or apple	Fennel tea
DAY 6		
Rice Krispies with chopped dried apricots, almonds and grapenuts	Asparagus with melted cheese	Baked herring with onions, mushrooms, sweetcorn and new potatoes
	Tomato and onion salad with basil and olive oil, black pepper	
Oat cakes with Whole Earth peanut butter	Grapefruit juice	Summer fruit pudding with fromage frais
Rooibosch tea	Pomelo	Raspberry and Ginseng tea
DAY 7		
Cheese omelette	Chickpea dip with raw carrot, broccoli and celery, poppadums, mung beans and alfalfa with walnut oil and lemon dressing	Turkey casserole
Wholemeal toast		Carrots, parsnips, sweet potato, peas, mashed potatoes
Orange marmalade	Pineapple juice	Fresh dates and pineapple
Barley Cup	Fresh blackberries	Lemon Verbena tea

Part Two
Healthy Pregnancy

CHAPTER 8

Pregnancy: Your Questions Answered

Q: *Will I need to eat more when I am pregnant, and if so what?*

A: Despite the fact that many of us feel like 'human vacuum cleaners' during pregnancy, the demand for calories does not rise significantly in the first six months of pregnancy, and only by an additional 10–20 per cent during the last three months of pregnancy. What *does* increase is the need for good quality foods which contain specific nutrients including folic acid, Vitamin B12, and the minerals zinc and iron. Slim woman may, however, experience a larger increase in calorie requirements earlier in their pregnancy.

As well as eating your three meals per day during pregnancy, at some stage you will probably feel the need to have a light mid-morning snack and perhaps another snack between your lunch and your evening meal. Try to choose good quality snacks like fruit, nuts, seeds, natural yoghurts, Ryvita and spreads like peanut butter or banana, or an oat, fruit and nut bar like the Jordan's Fruesli bars. By eating wholesome food regularly you will keep your blood sugar levels in an optimum range and feel less like attacking the biscuit tin!

Q: *Is it advisable to take iron supplements throughout pregnancy?*

A: Whilst some doctors routinely give iron supplements to women during pregnancy, the case for so doing appears to be weak, unless the individual has low iron levels or is a vegetarian. Although the demand for iron by the growing baby and placenta is considerably raised during pregnancy, we are actually conserving iron because we are no longer having monthly periods.

Women who have taken iron during pregnancy as part of clinical trials have reported very little benefit. In fact many of them experienced heartburn, constipation, diarrhoea or nausea. Consuming too much iron can upset the balance of other important nutrients like zinc, which is needed for the growth and development of the baby.

If you feel abnormally tired it would be advisable to ask your doctor to check your serum ferritin level, and only take iron supplements if it is found to be low. Make sure you consume a diet that is rich in foods containing iron, like green leafy vegetables, meat, beans, fortified-cereals, and eggs.

Q: *Is it necessary to take any vitamin or mineral supplements during pregnancy?*

A: In recent years folic acid has been shown to be vital in preventing three-quarters of neural tube defects (spina bifida). It is now recommended that all women who are planning to conceive take supplements which include 400 mcg of folic acid per day before conceiving. In addition to this, Vitamin B12 appears to work with folic acid reducing the chance of birth defects, so it would be advisable to take a daily supplement that has been specially designed for this purpose.

106

If you are eating an exceptionally healthy diet, which includes organic produce, and drinking very little tea, coffee or alcohol, then the chances are that you will be getting many of the nutrients that you need. However, if you are slight, a vegetarian, have an unplanned pregnancy, or have not been eating very well, then as a precaution it would be advisable to take a multi-vitamin and mineral supplement, *without* animal Vitamin A (retinol) each day anyway. It is far better to err on the side of caution.

Survey of 448 Mothers
SUPPLEMENTS TAKEN DURING THE LAST PREGNANCY

	Never	*Occasionally*	*Regularly*
Iron (doctor)	33.7%	20.0%	46.3%
Iron (purchased)	94.0%	3.8%	2.2%
Folic acid	45.5%	13.8%	40.7%
Multi-vitamins	79.5%	11.6%	8.9%
Vitamin B	94.2%	3.3%	2.5%
Evening primrose oil	97.1%	1.8%	1.1%

Q: *Are cravings during pregnancy a sign that you are lacking something?*

A: Women report cravings for all sorts of foods and drinks during their pregnancies, and often in the same woman no two pregnancies are alike in relation to their fancies. During my first pregnancy I managed to consume at least one or two pounds of herring roes per day, followed by melon of any description. In the second pregnancy it was parsley sauce, not just on fish, but on anything. The

107

third pregnancy was tart food like pickled herrings or lemons, and during the final pregnancy it was fizzy drinks. Were it not for the last pregnancy I would have said that all the foods craved were rich in folic acid, which is very important during the early stages of pregnancy. Sparkling water and tonic water blew my theory wide apart!

As far as I can gather, cravings for coal, washing powder and dirt are a result of a severe iron deficiency, but what lies behind fancies for food seem to be Mother Nature's secret. If your cravings happen to be for wholesome food there is no particular reason to curb them. However, if it's the chocolate bars or sweeties that have your attention, you would be wise to eat sweet dried fruit or fruit and nut bars instead.

Q: *Will drinking alcohol during pregnancy harm my growing baby?*

A: The alcohol that you drink during pregnancy is passed to your growing baby across the placenta *neat*. If the baby is exposed to excessive amounts of alcohol, brain damage and mental and growth retardation can result, as well as misformed facial features, and deformities of the heart and skeleton known as Foetal Alcohol Syndrome. Alcohol can also cause miscarriage, and certainly affects sperm production.

The most crucial times for the well-being of your eggs are prior to conception, at the time of fertilisation and during those first few weeks of development. As many of us don't realise we are pregnant until all of these stages have passed, it is advisable to stop drinking completely if you are even contemplating becoming pregnant. During the later stages of pregnancy the occasional glass of alcohol will probably not cause any damage, but by drinking regularly you are taking a great risk.

Q: *I smoke ten to fifteen cigarettes per day, should I cut down during pregnancy?*

A: It is advisable to stop smoking before becoming pregnant as part of your preconceptual programme. Tobacco smoke contains poisonous chemicals which are passed into your baby's bloodstream. Smoking can retard the growth of a developing baby, and increase your chances of miscarriage or premature birth. If you continue to smoke during pregnancy you are more likely to give birth to a baby with health problems like asthma and glue ear.

The optimum environment for both a growing baby and a new-born baby is smoke-free. If both you and your partner smoke, make a plan to give up together, so that you can support each other. Cutting down your cigarette consumption is not a satisfactory compromise, as you tend to inhale fewer cigarettes more deeply and as a result ingest the same amount of toxic chemicals. If you discover you are pregnant and you are still smoking, try to stop immediately as it will improve your chances of having a healthy baby.

Q: *Can I continue to drink coffee safely during pregnancy?*

A: During pregnancy women metabolise caffeine more slowly, and it is a stimulant which is passed across the placenta to the baby. In a mug of instant coffee there is approximately 100 mg of caffeine, whereas a mug of ground coffee contains up to 150 mg. Caffeine is also present in tea – one mug containing approximately 80–100 mg – cola-based drinks and, to a lesser degree, chocolate.

Research as to whether caffeine during pregnancy is actually harmful to the baby is inconclusive. To be safe

109

it is advisable to reduce your caffeine consumption and use alternative drinks. It just so happens that many women develop an aversion to coffee during pregnancy, which makes it all the easier to give up. See also page 80.

Q: *Do ultrasound scans have any effect on the unborn baby?*

A: Although we all like to see our growing baby wave at us on the scanning machine, because no trial has ever been conducted to assess the safety of ultrasound, doctors are suggesting that scans are only performed in circumstances where the information is likely to be useful. Frequent routine scanning throughout the pregnancy is not likely to be on offer as there is still a question mark as to whether ultrasound investigations in pregnancy may restrict the growth of the baby.

Although the Department of Health has found no cause for concern, following research in Australia they now only offer a scan to women when they are eighteen weeks' pregnant.

Q: *Is there anything I can do to prevent stretch marks from forming?*

A: Stretch marks occur more commonly in women who have pale skin, whereas women with olive skin or black skin seem to escape with few. The degree of elasticity of your skin also plays a part in determining whether or not you are left with stretch marks after pregnancy. There has been some suggestion that low zinc stores and possibly low levels of essential fatty acids may contribute to a predisposition to stretch marks.

When you consider how far the skin of your abdomen has to stretch it is not surprising that pregnancy sometimes leaves its mark. As well as taking a multi-vitamin and mineral pill each day, I always rubbed my tummy with Efamol evening primrose oil, which seemed to ease the skin tension.

Q: *What sort of exercise should I take during pregnancy?*

A: Keeping your body fit during pregnancy has a dual payback. Firstly you will be in better shape to deliver your baby. Secondly, the brain chemicals, endorphins, which are released as a result of low-impact aerobic exercise, improve your sense of well-being which, it seems, is passed on to your growing baby.

Research shows that if you are in good health it is safe to exercise in pregnancy. If you are fit when you become pregnant you can continue with your exercise routine until you feel you need to slow down in later pregnancy. If you haven't been exercising regularly then you will need to start gradually, perhaps with an exercise video at home. The YMCA produce an excellent pregnancy video called *Y Plan Before and After Pregnancy.*

In order to get your Vitamin D requirement you will need to take some regular exercise in daylight, and better still, in sunlight when it is available.

Q: *Is it important to have regular relaxation time during pregnancy and which are the best methods of relaxation?*

A: Being able to relax at will is often an acquired ability, but a very important skill, especially during pregnancy. Being in a relaxed state will help you to cope with your ante-natal checks and your labour, as well as helping to keep your blood pressure in the normal range. When you are expecting your first child it is far easier to find the time to relax. Having one or more little children to

111

deal with as well can easily result in your relaxation time being forgotten. Try to fit in your relaxation when they are sleeping, or get a relative or friend to watch them for a while so that you can have some uninterrupted time to yourself.

If you already practise yoga or meditation you will be able to continue with your twenty minutes or so each day. If you have thus far led a busy life and haven't had much quiet time, try to set aside half an hour each day to do some do-it-yourself relaxation. Take the phone off the hook, put on some soothing music, and lie in a comfortable position with your head supported by a cushion. Beginning with your feet, try to concentrate on each group of muscles, first tensing them, then relaxing them, gradually building your way up to your face. When you have completed this, lie still and let your mind wander into a pleasant day-dream. When you have finished, come around slowly, and sit up for a few minutes before you stand up. Relaxation will lower your blood pressure and if you attempt to get up too quickly you could feel quite dizzy.

You may well have many more questions about pregnancy and health. Do ask your general practitioner or health visitor. Some specialist organisations given in the Appendix on page 281 give useful information sheets or pamphlets, so do contact them. The WNAS can also help further with nutrition-related problems such as PMS and dietary difficulties.

CHAPTER 9

Potential Dangers During Pregnancy

As each year goes by, our planet becomes less and less like the Garden of Eden. Most of us are bombarded by small amounts of potentially harmful toxins and environmental pollution every day of our lives. There are petrol fumes in the air, pesticides on our food, pests *in* our food, toxins in our water and undesirable radiation from electric appliances. This doesn't even include irradiated food, the rays from microwaves, chemicals we use for cleaning our homes, the E numbers in our food, pet infections, or any occupational hazards we may encounter. It's a wonder we are all still standing.

Prior to the thalidomide disaster of the 1960s, it was assumed that the placenta protected the growing baby from toxins that its mother consumed or encountered. A drug that seemed safe in pregnant animals was assumed to be safe for consumption by pregnant women, but when thousands of babies were born with deformities the world had to think again. Understandably doctors and prospective parents alike have taken a far more cautious approach when considering drug options ever since.

According to official figures the percentage of babies born with birth defects has been pretty steady for some time – between 3 and 5 per cent. Whilst many of these deformed babies suffer with genetic problems or chromosomal damage, one in ten is thought to be attributable to environmental causes.

As there is no greener planet awaiting us, we have to make the most of what we have. There are many things that we can do for ourselves that will improve our environment, and subsequently improve the chances of a healthy life for our children. So many pregnancies are unplanned, which means that life-long damage could have already been done by the time a woman discovers that she is pregnant. It would make great sense to clean up your environment and improve your diet for the sake of your own health whether you were planning a baby or not. The motivation to make changes has probably never been greater, so let us look at some of the areas you should be concentrating on.

At Home	Our Food	External Factors
household chemicals	bugs and bacteria	X rays
pets and pet chemicals	irradiated food	nuclear power
tap water	pesticides	occupational risks
microwave ovens	additives	electric cables
	E numbers	sunlight
	toxic metals	

At Home

You may never have really stopped to think about the number of chemicals that you come into regular contact with inside your own home. We have discovered that the growing baby does not have a sufficiently mature system to deal with toxins, especially in the early stages of development. As it seems that many of the toxins you come into contact with will find their way across the placenta to the baby, it makes sense to be aware and limit the use of chemicals where possible.

★ Oven cleaners are usually pretty toxic, so there has never been a better excuse to get someone else to clean your oven. Failing that, just use an all-purpose cleaner and a little more elbow grease!

★ Pet sprays are often pretty lethal too, especially the flea sprays, which should be avoided completely from the time you decide to conceive onwards.

★ Fly sprays, which you may not have thought twice about, must be pretty potent as they kill flies. Use a fly swatter instead.

★ Paint contains many chemicals, even if it is lead-free. If you are planning to decorate your house, do it before you start your preconceptual programme, or go away for a few days whilst the paint smell is still in the air.

★ Solvents which contain substances like benzene are thought to be associated with increased risk of cancer, and are considered harmful to a growing baby.

★ The quality of tap water varies depending upon where you live. In an ideal world clean tap water is good for us as it contains many useful trace elements. Sadly many water supplies are contaminated with nitrates and toxic metals like lead, so it may be advisable to use a water filter, making sure that you change the filter regularly. Your local water authority should be able to give you details about the levels of undesirable substances in your water supply.

★ The committee are still out on the subject of microwave ovens. There is no argument that microwaves do change the structure of cells, and it is thought that they may well cause harm to our growing infants. While the debate goes on it is probably safer to avoid the microwave where possible and use alternative methods of cooking.

PETS

Although we love our pets, and they may appear to be clean, they may carry bugs which could harm your unborn baby. When the baby is born, no matter how close you are to your pets, they will naturally take second place. They should eat and sleep in a separate area, and all their belongings should be kept apart from yours.

★ Keep pets out of the kitchen where possible, and do not allow them to walk on kitchen work-surfaces.

★ Prepare their pet food in a separate place from your own food preparation, and keep their utensils and bowls separate.

★ Wash pet bowls and utensils thoroughly with their own washing-up brush and dry them with their own tea-towel.

★ If you have a cat that has a litter tray, whilst you are pregnant get someone else to change the litter for you preferably every twenty-four hours (see also page 121).

★ Always wash your hands after handling or stroking your pet.

★ Soil in the garden may have been contaminated by cats. It is worth taking the precaution of wearing gloves for gardening, and washing your hands thoroughly when you remove the gloves.

★ Toxoplasma is a rare disease that can cause miscarriage. It is contracted following contact with sheep and new-born lambs. Simply don't go anywhere near sheep when you are pregnant, especially in the lambing season.

OUR FOOD

Analysing what happens to much of our food before it gets to the table can be a pretty off-putting experience. But unless you are self-sufficient, which most of us are not, it is a question of becoming familiar with the options and getting the balance right. In order to do this we need to look at how our food is grown, what changes are made to it, what is added to it before it reaches the shops, and what can infect it.

THE GROWING PROCESS

Much of our vegetables, fruit and grains are grown in soil that contains potentially harmful chemicals which, in large quantities, could damage your growing baby.

Nitrates present in the soil either come from animal manure or plant debris, or from nitrogen-containing fertilisers designed to increase the crop yield. They can reduce the supply of oxygen available to your baby, known as blue baby syndrome, and have been associated with stomach cancer. Breast-fed babies are relatively protected from nitrates as the mother's body screens them out before they get to the milk.

Our crops are often sprayed with pesticides and insecticides which makes a richer harvest at the expense of our health. Their aim is to kill off undesirable life forms which they do successfully, but it seems their poisons have detrimental effects on humans too. Some researchers have shown that these apparently safe substances affect the growing baby, particularly the nervous system, the developing spinal cord and the liver.

The over-use of chemicals in the long term interferes with mineral balance in the soil, and the result is abundant crops that contain fewer nutrients than nature intended. The Soil Association lobbies hard to reverse the policy to chemicalise our food, but it remains a highly political issue.

The interim solution is to wash all vegetables and fruit thoroughly, and where possible to buy organic produce, which has not been chemically treated or grown in chemically treated soil. Unless you grow your own it does cost more, but you will have to weigh up whether chemical-free food containing more nutrients is worth that bit extra.

FOOD ADDITIVES

Whilst there are some perfectly harmless substances added to food, the number of potentially harmful additives is significant. Many additives have been shown to cause hyperactivity in children, asthma, eczema, skin rashes and swelling. It is obviously important to be able to differentiate between the safe and not-so-safe additives, rather than assuming that all additives are bad. For example Vitamin B2, riboflavin, is used as a yellow colouring agent, and Vitamin C, L-Ascorbic, is used as a preservative.

IRRADIATED FOOD

The process of irradiating food was introduced to increase the shelf life of food, which it does successfully. The gamma rays kill microscopic bacteria, but also alter the composition of the food, depleting and sometimes destroying many of the important vitamins, including folic acid. Whilst irradiation may make food last longer, it prevents it from looking or smelling bad even when it is. The result is that we could easily be fooled into eating food that is unfit for consumption. The British Medical Association is firmly opposed to food irradiation, and most of the large supermarkets have refused to stock irradiated food. If you are concerned, do check with your local supermarket, as by law irradiated food does not have to be labelled so.

It is sad to realise that the root of most of the decisions that are made to tamper with our food supply are economically motivated. Were our health the prime concern there would undoubtedly be rapid changes in farming policies. Until then we have to fend for ourselves.

TOXIC METALS

Toxic metals have a detrimental effect on fertility and the growing baby, so it is important to avoid foods that have been contaminated.

★ Don't go berry picking at the roadside or have a picnic in a car park, as lead levels are likely to be high.

★ Avoid using tins of food, like tuna, when the tin does not have a plastic inner lining as the food may have very high lead levels.

★ Make sure your water supply does not come through old lead piping.

★ Avoid consuming processed foods, which are high in cadmium, another toxic metal, as the refining process increases the cadmium ratio.

★ Don't have any more mercury fillings in your teeth. Better still, have the old ones removed six months before you are planning to conceive, as it is very toxic to our growing babies who receive it in great concentration through the placenta.

★ Avoid saucepans or baking dishes that are made from aluminium as this metal has been associated with behaviour disorders and an increased incidence of Alzheimer's disease, amongst other things.

★ Don't use copper pans either, as high levels of copper have also been shown to be harmful to the growing baby and are thought to produce behaviour disorders in children. As women have naturally higher levels of copper during pregnancy, they have no need for a further top-up.

BUGS AND BACTERIA

It is all too easy during pregnancy to come into contact with germs that can harm your unborn baby. Keeping a clean and ordered home will help, but there are danger situations that may be occurring in your environment without your knowledge Raw meat, eggs, soft cheese and pâté may be the source of harmful bacteria. It is important to be aware of the hazards so that you can organise a way of avoiding contact with these undesirables.

You may have heard various technical words used to describe some of these unwelcome bacteria like listeriosis, Salmonella or toxoplasmosis, and justifiably wondered what they were. Their names are not exactly user-friendly or descriptive.

Listeriosis

This is a flu-like illness which is caused by the bug, Listeria monocytogenes. It is found in some common foods which should be avoided during pregnancy, as even a mild dose can cause miscarriage, severe illness in a new-born baby, or even a still-birth. The types of foods that contain Listeria are:

★ soft cheeses like Camembert, Brie, Roquefort, Stilton and other blue-veined cheeses
★ unpasteurised cheese or dairy products including goat and sheep products
★ liver pâté of any type
★ cook-chill meals. These are ready-cooked, and kept cold, but not frozen, and are designed to be eaten cold or to be reheated at home. As many of these meals, including ready-to-eat poultry, contain small amounts of Listeria, it is advisable to avoid them altogether or to cook them until they are extremely hot
★ undercooked meat of any description
★ pre-prepared salads
★ soft ice-cream from a machine
★ food that is past its best-before date

Salmonella

This is a bacteria responsible for more food poisoning than any other. Once contaminated, you are likely to experience

120

symptoms of sickness and diarrhoea. Poultry and eggs are probably the most common foods to be contaminated with Salmonella, but thorough cooking often eliminates the bug. Despite precautions approximately one in twenty eggs contains Salmonella.

★ Don't eat anything that contains raw or uncooked egg, and don't forget less obvious foods like mousse and mayonnaise.
★ Only eat eggs that have been cooked so thoroughly that the egg yolk is hard.
★ Always wash your hands thoroughly if you have been touching raw meat, especially poultry.
★ Don't let raw meat come into contact with any other food. This includes any spillage that may occur in the fridge.
★ Use a special board to prepare meat and poultry, which is kept only for that purpose. Scrub it very thoroughly with hot water after use, and do the same with any surface touched.
★ Cook all meat and poultry thoroughly so that the bacteria are destroyed.

Toxoplasmosis
This is again a flu-like illness, which is caused by an infection by the bug called Toxoplasma gondii, sometimes found in raw meat, especially lamb, and also in cat faeces. As it can affect the unborn child it is important to take precautions.

★ Never eat undercooked or raw meat.
★ Wash your hands thoroughly after preparing meats.
★ Wash all food preparation surfaces with very hot water or bleach.
★ Clean and scrub all vegetables thoroughly to ensure that all soil and dirt is removed. If cats have soiled the earth, our food can be contaminated.

★ Don't let your cat have kittens at the time you plan to be pregnant, as kittens carry toxoplasmosis.
★ Clear up cat mess with boiling water or bleach.

Unpasteurised milk
Milk that has not been heat-treated may therefore contain bugs that are harmful to our health. Avoid 'green top' unpasteurised, or any milk that has not been heat-treated, from the time you start to plan your baby, until you have finished breast-feeding.

EXTERNAL FACTORS

As if there were not enough dangers in the home and in the food that we buy, external factors – power cables, radiation, even sunlight – can all be potentially harmful to our unborn babies.

RADIATION
Background radiation is something that we are constantly bumping into in life, very often without even knowing it. Radios, televisions, microwave ovens, satellite systems and VDUs all pump out small doses of rays on a regular basis. Our bodies can and do deal with a certain amount of radiation, and indeed eating a nutritious diet aids this process.

At higher doses, though, radiation may be extremely damaging and even life-threatening. There is a high incidence of leukaemia in those who live near or work at the Sellafield nuclear power plant in the UK, and following the Chernobyl disaster in the USSR in 1987 there has been a high incidence of cancer reported in both adults and children.

When planning a pregnancy, it makes sense to keep away from major sources of radiation. If you live near a nuclear plant, consider moving, and if you work in one, consider changing your job.

If you need an X ray either during your preconceptual phase or pregnancy, let your carers know that you are planning a pregnancy or that you have already conceived. If you had an X ray before you knew you were pregnant go along to discuss the situation with your doctor. Avoid dental X rays as well.

POWER CABLES

A relatively recent discovery is that people living within 500 metres (550 yds) of an overhead power line are more prone to symptoms of fatigue, palpitations, eye pain and constant noises in the ear, so much so that the Central Electricity Generating Board launched a £500,000 study into the effects of high-voltage power cables on our health. There is concern amongst some researchers that the electromagnetic fields emitted by these power lines could be responsible for causing birth defects and even cancer in the offspring of those who have lived or worked in close proximity. Until studies provide us with conclusive evidence, it is advisable to keep your distance.

OCCUPATIONAL RISKS

Whilst some of the occupational hazards that we face are well publicised, like repetitive strain injury, the effects of poor ventilation and lighting, and many other more far-reaching consequences of doing our job, are often overlooked. Between 1980 and 1982 the Office of Population Censuses and Surveys conducted a survey on people in England and Wales, looking specifically at the effects of certain occupations on reproduction. There were some surprising findings.

★ Road transport drivers had more risk of having a baby

with Down's syndrome, deformities of the central nervous system, a cleft palate or cardiovascular disease, presumably because of their frequent contact with lead from petrol and other exhaust fumes.

★ Textile workers had higher rates of still-born babies or babies that died shortly after birth, which is presumably related to industrial fumes.

★ Petroleum process plant operators had children with more congenital deformities, again as a result of inhaled fumes.

★ Welders were found to have a high incidence of spina bifida children and sudden infant death.

★ Publicans had more babies with cleft palate deformities, which is thought to be due to their alcohol consumption and hours spent in a smoky environment.

Other studies have shown the following:

★ Nurses working in operating theatres have more deformed children than nurses working in other areas of a hospital, probably due to their close contact with anaesthetic gases.

★ Female anaesthetists had twice as many deformed babies as other female doctors.

★ Female dental surgeons have high rates of miscarriage, possibly from regular contact with a combination of anaesthetic and mercury.

Offices have their share of hazards too, the most researched of which is the consequences of sitting too long in front of the screen of a visual display unit, VDU. One study has shown that working with a VDU for more than twenty hours per week during the first three months of pregnancy is likely to double the risk of miscarriage. Although many studies have suggested that working with

124

a VDU increases the risk of infertility, miscarriage and deformity, large studies in Scandinavia and Canada have failed to find a similar association.

Whilst the research remains inconclusive you will have to make your own decisions about VDUs. When you sit down to work on a VDU an electro-magnetic field is formed, and you can expect to be on the receiving end of small amounts of radiation. In view of this it is probably wise to limit your time on the VDU and to take regular breaks when you are working with it.

SUNLIGHT

There are definite pros and cons about sunlight, and so it is very much a question of getting the balance right. The sun provides us with natural light, it breathes life into our vegetation, kills infection and gives us a psychological boost. However, the sun's rays in large doses can cause cancer, and with our increased exposure to these rays due to the thinning of the ozone layer, it is advisable to limit the time you spend in the hot sun.

The best plan of action is to take regular exercise in the open when the heat of the day has passed. That way you get the therapeutic effect of the sun without getting an excess helping of harmful rays.

Learning to make the most of your environment is an acquired skill that many of us learn as we go along. We may not live in a perfect world, but we do have choices. If we each take responsibility for cleaning up our immediate environment and do a little campaigning along the way, we are much more likely to live to enjoy our happy, healthy children.

CHAPTER 10

Diet for Pregnancy

During pregnancy and breast-feeding, the female body has a higher need for vitamins, minerals and other essential nutrients than at any other time. Besides your own body, there are the needs of a growing baby to consider, as well as the increased tissue of the uterus, placenta and blood. All this new tissue requires more calories, proteins, vitamins and minerals.

During pregnancy there is a demand for calorie intake to be increased by an additional 10–20 per cent, as energy requirements vary considerably from woman to woman. It is normal to gain nearly 12.5 kg (27.6 lb) in weight during pregnancy, but weight gain can be from 6.3–19 kg (1–3 stones, 14–42 lb). Metabolic rates vary, so whilst some women will hardly notice a change in appetite, others will feel like eating for two or more! Studies have shown that women who gain in excess of 13.5 kg (30 lb) during pregnancy have more healthy babies, with slim women with only small weight gain having babies who have low birth weights.

Approximately 3–3.6 kg (7–8 lb) of this new weight will be the baby, and the remainder will be the increased tissue weight of the uterus, placenta, blood and fat stores. The fat stores are particularly useful during breast-feeding as they are converted into breast-milk. Thin women are less likely to be able to give their babies all the nutrients they need, so don't get too conscious about the extra pounds during pregnancy, and never diet unless you are grossly overweight, and then only diet under supervision. If you are eating a healthy diet and taking regular exercise, you will find the extra pounds will disappear naturally in the months following the birth of your baby.

WHAT'S IN SHORT SUPPLY

If your diet only just provides adequate levels of certain nutrients, a deficiency state may exist during or towards the end of the pregnancy. For example, it is routine now for your doctor to do tests for anaemia in the early part of the pregnancy, and give supplements of iron as a preventative measure. Folic acid deficiency is now clearly linked to neural tube defects and so it is advisable for every woman to take 400 mcg of folic acid per day, from the time she decides to conceive, right through until at least the end of the first trimester of pregnancy.

Deficiency of other vitamins and minerals has also been associated with problems during pregnancy. The trace mineral zinc is important in growth and development, and deficiency in the mother during pregnancy has been linked to low birth weights, under 2.72 kg (6 lb). Additionally, a good intake of B vitamins during the early stages of pregnancy is associated with a better outcome. Vitamin A is another nutrient linked to growth, and in fact it has long been recommended by the Department of Health that all pregnant and breast-feeding mothers take supplements of Vitamins A as beta-carotene, D and C in order to build up vitamin stores that can be passed across the placenta and through the breast-milk to the growing baby. These supplements should be taken by those who are not eating well, have a poor intake of fresh fruit and vegetables, and those at risk of Vitamin D deficiency. They are provided free to those on Income Support in the UK.

All of these nutrients are essential for the baby's growth during pregnancy. The placenta assists in the exchange of nutrients between the mother's blood and the growing baby's circulation, as it literally pumps vitamins from the mother to the infant. Mother Nature has designed it so that the baby gets the pick of the nutrients and it is mother herself who gets left 'high and dry' when there is a shortage. In fact, your general health in the latter stages of pregnancy, and rate of recovery from delivery, is very much influenced by your overall health and the quality of your diet during the pregnancy. The picture is appearing that the mother's diet before conceiving, and in the early part of the pregnancy, particularly affects the baby. Whereas the diet during the pregnancy and after is a main determinant of the mother's health at the end of pregnancy and after delivery.

In the last four to six weeks of pregnancy, the baby is rapidly storing essential vitamins and minerals ready for the first few weeks and months of life. Premature infants who have not had the opportunity to set aside stores of essential nutrients, or those whose mums were under-nourished, are particularly predisposed to certain nutritional deficiencies, infections, and the prospect of having increased chances of contracting heart disease, stroke, high cholesterol and blood pressure levels and diabetes later on in life.

Survey of 448 Mothers
DIET DURING THE LAST PREGNANCY

	No reply	None	Daily	Most days	Once or twice weekly	Occasionally
Breakfast	4	15	296	90	5	38
Fortified cereals	7	92	175	99	14	61
Cooked main meal	1	11	305	111	9	11
Liver pâté/ liver	2	415	1	2	4	24
Soft cheese	3	419	1	3	4	18
Hard cheese	1	66	53	104	109	115
Chocolate	2	19	103	133	83	108
Eggs – not hard-boiled	1	276	4	13	48	106
Meat	1	33	124	188	71	31
Fish	1	74	24	62	138	149
Chicken	2	34	38	107	175	92

15 women out of our sample never had breakfast, and 11 did not eat a cooked meal. 31 women whose babies were under age 15 months were eating liver and liver pâté; 26 women were eating soft cheese; and 171 women were eating eggs that were not hard-boiled. 33 women did not eat meat, 74 never ate fish, 34 did not eat chicken, although there were 16 vegetarians in the sample

129

and no vegans. 103 women ate chocolate daily and a further 133 had chocolate most days. On a more positive note, 175 women ate fortified cereals daily, and a further 99 had fortified cereals most days.

WHAT TO CHOOSE

You should have a good appetite during pregnancy, apart from some morning sickness in the first three or four months (see page 158 for some helpful tips). You should be eating enough to gain weight at the rate of 225–450 g (½–1lb) per week, unless you are overweight.

★ **Eat a wide variety of nutritious foods** The best are those foods rich in protein, such as lean meat (preferably additive-free), fish, free-range chicken, nuts, seeds, peas, beans and lentils.

Certain foods are particularly nutritious in their content of Vitamin B, iron and other trace minerals, the requirements of which increase substantially during pregnancy. They include:
* lean meat
* eggs, preferably free-range
* all green vegetables
* wheatgerm
* nuts
* wholemeal bread (up to three slices per day)
* fortified breakfast cereal

Make sure you include a selection of these in your diet on a regular basis.

★ **Choose vegetable rather than animal fats** Go for

polyunsaturated margarines and cold pressed oils, rather than animal fats which are high in calories and low in essential nutrients. You need to fill up with the best quality food you can lay your paws on! Cut any visible fat off meat and poultry, including the skin.

★ **Ensure you have a good intake of calcium** Dairy products such as cheese, milk and yoghurt are all good sources of calcium, as are bony fish like tinned sardines, nuts, seeds, and green vegetables. They also provide protein and other nutrients. Consume 300–600 ml (½–1 pint) of milk and yoghurt per day, and 175–225 g (6–8 oz) of cheese per week.

★ **Eat plenty of salad, vegetables and fruit** You should have a good portion of fresh green leafy vegetables or salad daily, plus at least two portions of fresh fruit. These are an important source of vitamins, minerals and fibre.

★ **Be sensible about sweet foods** May women during pregnancy develop a craving, an appetite for sugary and sweet foods. This is allowable, but only provided that you are already eating a well-balanced and nutritious diet. A portion of dessert or a small amount of chocolate at the end of a meal will certainly do no harm, provided that you had a good intake of nutritious foods in the main part of the meal. Cakes, biscuits and puddings mean loads of calories and hardly any nutrients, so if you are prone to weight gain, you should eat fruit instead, or choose desserts with a fruit base.

★ **Drink fruit juice instead of tea with your meals** Iron is a particularly important nutrient during pregnancy as your baby will be stocking up on iron to last through the first few months of life. Tea contains tannin which binds with iron from vegetable proteins and reduces the amount that is absorbed into the body. However, if you drink a glass of orange juice, which is high in Vitamin C, you will double the amount of iron available to both you and

your baby. Other drinks high in Vitamin C are grapefruit, blackcurrant and tomato juices. Foods containing
high levels of Vitamin C include citrus fruits like oranges,
grapefruits and lemons, blackcurrants, strawberries, red
peppers, tomatoes and raw green vegetables.

★ **Drink tea and coffee alternatives** Rooibosch Eleven
O'Clock Tea is a caffeine-free tea look-alike, available from
health-food shops. In fact trials have shown that this tea
helps to soothe colic in young babies. There are many
varieties of herbal tea available to try, some fruity and
some which taste of herbs and spices like fennel or ginger.
You will need to experiment a bit until you find the teas
that appeal to your palate. Fortunately these days health-
food shops sell single sachets, so that you can sample
them before committing yourself to a whole box.

Barley Cup is a cereal drink that resembles coffee.
Dandelion coffee comes either instant, which is sweet,
or as dandelion root which you can boil or put through a
coffee filter. It tastes like a stronger malted drink. Chicory
is another coffee look-alike, which is an acquired taste.

★ **Take adequate daily exercise** Exercising regularly will
keep you healthy, tone your muscles for the delivery, and
will provide your baby with a happier environment.
Research shows that low-impact aerobic exercise, three
or four times per week, encourages the brain to release
chemicals called endorphins, which raise your mood and
give you a 'buzz'. It is now thought that these endorphins
cross the placenta and give the baby a share of your
increased sense of well-being! For further ideas about
the kind of exercise to embark on, see Chapter 12.

SAMPLE MENUS FOR LATER PREGNANCY AND BREAST-FEEDING

DAY ONE
Breakfast
Cornflakes with Grapenuts, raisins, chopped almonds, banana, Bio Yoghurt and milk, wholemeal toast and marmalade
Rooibosch tea

Mid-morning snack
Jordan's Fruesli Bar
Glass of milk

Lunch
Sardines and mixed salad with walnut oil and lemon dressing
Ryvita
Orange juice
Fresh pear

Mid-afternoon snack
Slice of carrot cake or flap-jack
Dandelion coffee

Dinner
Turkey and vegetable curry with brown rice, mango chutney and poppadoms
Lychees and ice-cream

Grapefruit juice and ginger ale

DAY TWO
Breakfast
Wholemeal pancakes with stewed fruit filling
Fresh orange

Mid-morning snack
Bio Yoghurt with chopped fruit
Rooibosch tea

Lunch
Broccoli and cauliflower cheese
Jacket potato
Pineapple juice
Fresh dates

Mid-afternoon snack
Jordan's Fruesli bar
Barley Cup

Dinner
Mackerel in egg and lemon sauce, new potatoes, green beans and cauliflower
Pancakes with mixed berries and crème fraîche
Dandelion coffee

DAY THREE
Breakfast
Scrambled eggs with tomatoes and mushrooms
Ryvita and marmalade
Dandelion coffee

Mid-morning snack
Oatcakes with Whole Earth mixed nut butter
Barley Cup

Lunch
Artichoke with vinaigrette dressing
Walnut, sweetcorn and red pepper salad
Strawberries and raspberries with *fromage frais*
Pink grapefruit juice

Mid-afternoon snack
Scone with jam and cream
Glass of milk

Dinner
Peppered steak with jacket potato, mushrooms, sweetcorn and Brussels sprouts
Banana and cinnamon tea

DAY FOUR
Breakfast
Jordan's Oat Crunchy cereal with almonds and chopped dried apricots, Bio Yoghurt and milk
Toast and Whole Earth peanut butter
Rooibosch tea

Mid-morning snack
Fresh apple
Pineapple juice

Lunch
Pilchards in tomato sauce with chopped asparagus, mung beans and watercress salad
Satsumas
Orange and raspberry juice

Mid-afternoon snack
Oatcakes with Whole Earth fruit spread
Raspberry and ginseng tea

Dinner
Nut roast with baked parsnips, swede, sweet potato and broccoli
Dandelion coffee

DAY FIVE
Breakfast
Orange juice
Rice Crispies with raisins, chopped pear, pecan nuts and sunflower seeds, Bio

Yoghurt and milk
Oatcakes with apple and pear spread
Rooibosch tea

Mid-morning snack
Raw carrot and celery with hummus
Pink grapefruit juice

Lunch
Avocado with walnut and lemon dressing
Fennel, alfalfa, mung beans and red pepper salad
Tomato juice
Pomelo or orange

Mid-afternoon snack
Date and walnut loaf
Barley Cup

Dinner
Watercress soup
Pasta bake with tuna, walnuts and black olives
Green salad
Fresh fruit salad
Decaffeinated coffee

DAY SIX
Breakfast
Muesli with Grapenuts, almonds, sliced banana, Bio Yoghurt and milk

Toast with marmalade
Dandelion coffee

Mid-morning snack
Ryvita with Whole Earth peanut butter
Rooibosch tea

Lunch
Fried cod's roe with coleslaw
New potato salad
Orange juice
Pear and raisins

Mid-afternoon snack
Cheese cubes and walnuts
Glass of milk

Dinner
Stir-fry shrimps and squid with seaweed, snow peas and baby sweetcorn
Egg noodles
Fruit compote with custard
Raspberry and ginseng tea

DAY SEVEN
Breakfast
Grapefruit juice
Poached eggs with tomatoes and mushrooms
Ryvita and Whole Earth fruit spread
Rooibosch tea

135

Mid-morning snack
Fresh banana
Glass of milk

Mid-afternoon snack
Oat flapjack
Lemon verbena tea

Lunch
Root vegetable soup
Corn on the cob with mixed
  salad
Fresh pineapple and logan-
  berries

Dinner
Roast lamb with roast
  potatoes, carrots, cabbage,
  baked onions, spinach and
  redcurrant jelly
Baked stuffed apples
Mixed berry tea

CHAPTER 11

Screening Options During Pregnancy

Although childbirth is no longer associated with the enormous risks of past centuries, there are still things that can go wrong in a minority of cases. Generally our bodies are designed to produce normal healthy children and, with a little modern intervention, most of us do. If you consider yourself to be healthy with no hereditary problems in your family, you may not feel the need for serious intervention during your pregnancy. As some of the tests available carry with them risks of miscarriage, you will need to carefully weigh up the pros and cons before making a decision about individual tests.

Women under 35 are unlikely to be offered many of the tests available unless they are particularly at risk. As our ovaries age, our chances of making babies with deformities increase. At the age of 25 it is estimated that only one in 1,500 women is at risk of having a Down's syndrome baby, for instance. At 30 the chances increase to one woman in 800 and by 35 the chances are one in 300. By the age of 40 you are down to a one in 100 chance and at 45 a one in 30 chance. So you can see how the ageing process affects the quality of our eggs.

The theory behind modern screening during pregnancy is that early detection of major deformities and subsequent termination will lower the number of deformed babies born.

Having an early termination will also mean that you will not have to make the major life adjustment necessary for bringing up a mentally or physically disadvantaged child.

Many of the modern tests will show whether your baby is likely to have spina bifida or Down's syndrome. If you have a family history of one of these problems the chances are that you will welcome the test, regardless of the associated risk. However, if you would be against terminating your pregnancy, even if your baby was found to be deformed, then you may feel that screening during pregnancy is undesirable.

No matter where you stand regarding screening at the moment, it is important to know what each test has to offer as well as the risks associated with it, so that you can make an informed choice. Let's take a look at what's on offer.

ULTRASOUND

The ultrasound scan is used at some stage in most pregnancies these days. It is a system of using ultrasonic sound waves which are beamed on to the growing baby, and return signals are then transmitted via a computer into a visual image. The ultrasound scan is useful for detection of abnormalities like ectopic pregnancy – where the baby begins to grow in the fallopian tubes, instead of the uterus – deformed organs and some cases of neural tube defect. It is also an excellent way of detecting multiple pregnancies, assessing the growth of the developing child, and the position of the placenta. From as early as six or seven weeks the heartbeat of a live baby will be picked up by the ultrasound.

Understandably, this relatively new technology has created great excitement in medical circles, and indeed it has been popular with prospective parents, as they are actually able to see their babies on a computer screen. Some machines are even capable of producing a print of your baby in the uterus, which will no doubt have pride of place in the family album.

Although some clinics were using ultrasound routinely at regular intervals during pregnancy, current thinking is that a little more caution should be used, as the long-term side-effects of ultrasound scanning have yet to be fully assessed. Believe it or not, no trial has ever been conducted to test the safety of ultrasound, and some researchers believe that routine scanning may inhibit the baby's growth, and may even increase the incidence of leukaemia in exposed children.

The results of a study conducted in Australia have caused the Australians to rethink their scanning policy. They now only routinely conduct one scan at approximately eighteen weeks. The Department of Health in the UK remains unconcerned about long-term effects of scanning, but it would seem prudent to only use scanning when it will produce necessary information, and not just to say 'hello' to your baby. The view of the Consumers' Association is that 'Women who are offered a routine scan should be informed not only why it is recommended, but also that it is not an essential part of their antenatal care'.

ALPHA-FETOPROTEIN TEST (AFP)

This is a blood test that is usually performed at around sixteen weeks and measures alpha-fetoprotein, a protein manufactured in the baby's liver, which then crosses into the mother's bloodstream.

A raised level of AFP can indicate that your baby has a neural tube defect, when it will be suggested that you have an amniocentesis, or it could mean that you are having twins or that you are more pregnant than you thought you were, which can then be assessed by ultrasound.

There is no risk to mother or baby with this test, and the results take about a week to analyse. It is a valuable tool, but is not considered to be a conclusive test by itself.

THE BART'S TEST – MATERNAL SERUM SCREENING

This is my favourite test, which not only assesses your chances of having a baby with Down's syndrome, spina bifida or anencephaly (an absence of the higher part of the brain), but also has no side-effects! It is simply a triple blood test that was developed by Bart's Hospital in London, and is now offered routinely to all women in their catchment area. Some other areas around the country do offer it as an option, and failing that, your doctor or local hospital can arrange for you to receive the test privately.

This is a particularly important test if you are over the age of thirty-five, and therefore have increased chances of having a deformed baby. It cleverly assesses the actual age of your eggs, rather than their chronological age. So for example when I was tested during my last pregnancy, I was delighted to discover that the actual age of my eggs was equivalent to a woman ten years my junior at the time. My husband was delighted too, as he thought he had a 'new model'!

The Bart's test measures levels of alpha-fetoprotein which determine your risk of a neural tube defect and would be expected to be low in a woman carrying a Down's syndrome baby. It also measures a hormone called human chorionic gonadotrophin which is also likely to be high if you are carrying a Down's syndrome baby, and the hormone oestriol which would be expected to be low in the presence of Down's syndrome.

In order to achieve an accurate reading, the Bart's test has to be performed between the fifteenth and twenty-second week of pregnancy. If you have a positive result you will be strongly advised to have an amniocentesis. The only drawback with this test is that it is performed relatively late in pregnancy, and takes almost two weeks to analyse. If after amniocentesis you are then offered a termination, it is likely to be a very uncomfortable and distressing procedure, as by this time you are likely to be at least twenty weeks' pregnant.

AMNIOCENTESIS

This test is carried out at sixteen weeks, and is recommended for women over thirty-five, who have proved positive on the Bart's test, or for women who have a high risk of having a Down's syndrome baby or who have a family history of genetic problems like muscular dystrophy, chromosomal problems or haemophilia. The test is performed in hospital, but you will be allowed home shortly after. A hollow needle is inserted through the abdomen and into the fluid surrounding the baby, so that fluid containing cells can be drawn off for analysis. It is performed in conjunction with an ultrasound scan, so that the needle is kept away from the baby.

The risk of miscarriage after amniocentesis does increase slightly, and occasionally babies who move their limbs at the wrong time can be damaged. It is common to feel the uterus tightening after the test, and some women report feeling sore the next day. Women are usually advised to take it easy for a few days following the amniocentesis.

The value of amniocentesis is that it tests for spina bifida, muscular dystrophy and Down's syndrome. It can also reliably detect the sex of your baby. Apart from the discomfort and the small increased risk to your baby, the other drawback is that it takes four weeks for the result to come through. Although the alpha-fetoprotein results are available within a few days, the culture that is grown to assess chromosomal abnormalities takes much longer. The weeks of waiting can be agonising and unsettling, and once again if termination were suggested following a positive result you would be twenty weeks' pregnant. Having a pregnancy terminated so late can be psychologically disturbing as well as physically distressing.

CHORIONIC VILLUS SAMPLING (CVS)

This test involves removing by suction a small sample of the cells of the developing placenta, which can be done through the vagina or the wall of the abdomen. Like the amniocentesis it is performed in conjunction with an ultrasound scan. CVS will detect the same chromosomal abnormalities as amniocentesis, and genetic disorders such as sickle-cell anaemia and thalassaemia. It can also detect the sex of your baby. However, the developmental defects like spina bifida and neural tube defect are not within its remit.

The advantage of this test is that it is performed between the eighth and tenth week of pregnancy, and the results are usually through within a week to ten days. If termination were suggested following a positive result, you would probably be under twelve weeks' pregnant, in which case the experience would be less traumatic than the procedure following amniocentesis.

The disadvantages of CVS are as follows.

★ The incidence of miscarriage following CVS is further increased, depending on the skill of the surgeon. Figures quoted are in the 3 per cent range, but actual figures vary from study to study, and indicate that more miscarriages

occur in women who have had the CVS performed through the vagina, instead of through the abdomen.
★ There is a risk of infection to the baby as the amniotic sac surrounding the baby may be punctured.
★ The baby is exposed to a high dose of ultrasound.

Once again you will need to set aside a few days following the CVS to put your feet up. You may experience abdominal cramps, particularly if the sample is taken through the abdomen.

FETOSCOPY

A relatively new and wondrous procedure which involves inserting a microscopic camera into the uterus, so that the surgeon can check the baby for abnormalities like cleft palate or brain disorders. Whilst this test is usually a screening procedure which alerts doctors to the need for intensive care when the baby is born, babies can and are sometimes surgically treated before birth! They can have a complete blood transfusion whilst still in the uterus, and excess fluid could be drained, by means of a shunt, from the brain. These are obviously very skilled procedures that would at this time only be performed in a small number of specialist centres.

NEW TESTS

With the rapid advances in research of genetic disease it is possible to detect parents who may carry the gene for diseases such as cystic fibrosis. A test of the mother early in pregnancy could determine if she is a carrier; one in twenty of the normal population are. If so, testing her partner would identify those couples who run the risk of having a child with cystic fibrosis. If both are carriers the risk in any one offspring is one in four. Further assessment and termination might then be offered. Sophisticated tests that look for even rare genetically determined disease may well become routine in the future.

TERMINATION

If you disagree with termination you will never have to go through the soul-searching that obviously takes place in a woman who is contemplating termination. Making the decision to terminate a much wanted baby can be heartbreaking for both the expectant parents, and a period of bereavement is likely to take place. Having a late termination is even more complicated, as real labour very often has to take place, which must leave a woman physically and mentally crushed.

Taking advantage of any counselling on offer is sensible, and deciding to try for another baby as soon as it is advised would be a good plan. You will need a few months' breathing space though to get yourself back into good physical shape once your hormones have returned to normal, but research shows that your termination will not affect your future chances of becoming pregnant.

At the end of the day, once you have weighed up the pros and cons, don't forget that the choice is yours. It is *your* baby, and it is up to you to decide which tests you are prepared to have. Now that you are armed with the knowledge, taking into consideration your partner's views, you will be able to make an informed decision.

Chapter 12

The Value of Exercise

Exercise is not just a 'nice idea' if you can fit it into your busy schedule; it is vital to both your physical and mental well-being. It oxygenates your blood, stimulates the brain to release chemicals called endorphins which raise mood and energy levels, and has even been shown to offset the ageing of the central nervous system as well as protecting against heart disease.

Before Conceiving

Before pregnancy it is important to get yourself into the best possible all-round shape. No personal enhancement programme could be complete without a regular exercise routine.

★ You need to choose the type of exercise that you enjoy, and work out a schedule that will incorporate three or four sessions of aerobic exercise per week – swimming, brisk walking, running, dancing, playing squash, skipping or indeed doing an exercise work-out.
★ The length of time you spend exercising initially will depend upon your fitness level at the start. If you are reasonably fit you will need to aim for three or four

145

40-minute sessions of exercise per week, to the point of breathlessness. If you haven't been taking much exercise recently, then you will need to begin with just five or ten minutes four times per week, to the point of breathlessness, and build up gradually, over a period of weeks.

★ If you find it hard to motivate yourself at first, or to stick to your schedule, arrange to exercise with a friend, or make an appointment to attend a class where there is a financial penalty if you don't turn up!

★ When you work full-time it is not always easy to fit exercise into your work day. You will either have to make an early start in the mornings and exercise before you eat breakfast, or go to a class on your way home from work. If you do an exercise class after work you should eat a substantial snack an hour or two before setting off, to sustain you until dinner-time.

★ An exercise video to follow at home is always a good fall-back. The YMCA have an excellent range of videos which cover all fitness levels. Look out for their *Fitness Club* series. These work-outs are broken down into short comfortable sections which you can either do singly or incorporate two or three sections into your routine.

DURING PREGNANCY

Survey of 448 Mothers
EXERCISE

The average number of exercise sessions during pregnancy was between two and three per week.

Walking	89%
Swimming	34%

THE VALUE OF EXERCISE

Aerobics	6.2%
Aquafit	6.2%
Cycling	3.6%
Yoga	1.3%
Racquet sports	0.4%
Jogging	0.2%

Unless you are prone to miscarry, there is no reason why you shouldn't be able to continue with your exercise routine, at least for the first four or five months of pregnancy. There are some specialist classes for pregnancy which are worth looking out for, plus the YMCA have a video specifically to get you into shape during pregnancy, and back into shape, gradually, after the delivery.

Yoga classes for pregnancy are extremely beneficial and they help to make you more flexible. Once again there are special yoga poses for pregnancy, and in fact my yoga teacher Tricia Robinson made a video on yoga for pregnancy called *REP – Relaxation and Exercise in Pregnancy*. She used Cathy Taylor, the ex-athlete and morning TV presenter as her guinea pig, and I think it is well worth investing in.

Towards the end of your pregnancy you may find you prefer to concentrate on gentle exercise like yoga, walking and swimming. If you are a swimmer I really recommend a daily swim if you can manage it. I swam nearly every day during my pregnancies, and honestly feel it kept me going. Towards the end of pregnancy the swimming pool was the only place I felt comfortable. The water takes the weight of your baby, so that you no longer feel like a stranded whale. So much so, with my second baby I was tempted to stay in the pool when I felt the contractions start. I decided against it though, as I didn't fancy having a baby in cool water in public! I did have the next two in water though, which was a wonderful experience.

SHAPING UP AFTER PREGNANCY

Exercise will probably be the last thing on your mind when you have had the baby, but it is important to start doing your pelvic floor exercises whilst lying on the bed. Your midwife should give you a sheet about the basic exercises to do for the first few weeks, but it is sometimes hard to motivate yourself when there is so much else to do.

I found the exercise videos of immense help. There are specific exercises for the first few weeks after delivery, then you graduate to exercises designed for up to six weeks, and then from six weeks to four months. This means that you only do the exercises that your body should be doing at the appropriate stage. Some of the exercises are designed to be done with your baby, and you can certainly do the others with your baby by you in the crib or on a mat.

Pregnancy hormones affect both your joints and your ligaments, and it takes about four or five months for your body to physically return to its pre-pregnant state. Don't be impatient, take it day by day, and don't get disappointed by your lack of stamina.

WEIGHT LOSS

If you are one of those women who are able to wear your jeans the week after you have given birth, I hate you. Despite being slim initially, eating well and exercising, I always put on masses of weight during pregnancy. Post-natal exercise and breast-feeding helped to regain muscle tone after the birth, but it took me a full year each time to get back to my original weight, without dieting.

Don't be tempted to diet if you are breast-feeding. In my case it would have been impossible as when good food was in sight, I turned into a human vacuum cleaner! There will be plenty of time to get your figure back when you have stopped feeding, that is if you still have extra pounds. That excess fat does have a wonderful way of converting into breast-milk.

CHAPTER 13

The Benefits of Relaxation

Formal relaxation is an excellent method of warding off adverse stress from which we all suffer from time to time. When stress takes hold of us we not only feel uneasy, but it has a direct effect on our digestive process, and it is during times of great stress that people develop food intolerances. Severe stress has even been shown to suppress ovulation, which would be totally unacceptable whilst you are trying to conceive!

It's all very well for me to tell you to get twenty minutes' relaxation every day, but it's not always easy to switch off. Life in the 1990s can be very demanding and all-absorbing to the point where we don't naturally make time for ourselves. Some people have an amazing ability to switch off at will, whilst others find it extremely difficult to blot out the day-to-day stresses and demands. If you are one of the people who find it hard to let go, you may need to learn how to relax. There are several methods of relaxation ranging from yoga to self-hypnosis! So you will need to select a method and if necessary find an evening class to learn the technique.

Before you set off to get the prospectus for your local classes have a go at relaxing at home.

★ Wear some loose comfortable clothing, and make sure

the temperature of the room and the lighting are comfortable.
★ Put the answerphone on or take the phone off the hook.
★ Have some of your favourite music playing quietly in the background.
★ Place a pillow under your head.
★ Take a few slow deep breaths before you begin.
★ Concentrate on relaxing your muscles, starting with the toes on one foot and then the other. Gradually work your way slowly up your body, relaxing each group of muscles.
★ First tense each group of muscles, and then relax them, taking care to breathe deeply as you relax.
★ When you reach your head, and your face feels relaxed, remain in the relaxed position for about fifteen minutes.
★ When you feel the time is right gradually allow yourself to 'come to'. If you are happy with your relaxation technique, then aim to repeat it every day. Remember this is sacred time for you, when you shut out the world and concentrate on regenerating your batteries.

FORMAL RELAXATION METHODS

If you can't manage to switch off using this technique you will need to find a more formal method. There are at least a dozen recognised ways of formally relaxing, it is just a question of finding the one you enjoy the most.

YOGA
This discipline has been practised throughout the world for thousands of years. It works on the principle of bringing about a harmonious balance between your mind, body and soul. It is particularly effective at helping to relieve stress, and will tone your muscles at the same time. Apart from yoga classes, there are also suggested books on page 277

151

and yoga videos that you can watch at home.

CREATIVE VISUALISATION

This is my favourite method of distracting myself from the stresses of everyday life. It simply involves day-dreaming in a structured way. All you need to do is choose a scene that you would like to be part of – a favourite beach where you could dive with some dolphins, perhaps – and spirit yourself there in your imagination. You need to be lying down, with your eyes closed, in a warm and darkened environment, and then just let yourself float off. You will build up the ability to 'stay' there and not let your mind wander, as time goes by. When you come around you should feel warm, calm and relaxed, and maybe a little disappointed that you are not really in your day-dream!

SELF-HYPNOSIS

Self-hypnosis is a self-induced state that makes the mind susceptible to new ideas. When practised regularly it helps to bring about the feeling of calmness and mental agility. It is a system of implanting positive messages which have a therapeutic value and is thought to be particularly useful in helping to relieve stress, high blood pressure, migraine and insomnia. Some people find that it also helps them to overcome addictive habits. Half an hour each day can leave you feeling refreshed, relaxed and in a more positive mood.

MEDITATION

This is another way of separating you from your body, and has a calming and renewing effect on both mind and body. You will need to learn to meditate at a class, but once you have the skill you can use it any time, any place.

The beauty of all these techniques, and many others, is that they are very simple, cost very little, but are most beneficial.

If your partner is willing you should try out the techniques together, and compare notes.

Massage

No chapter on relaxation would be complete without singing the praises of massage, which is another wonderfully therapeutic way of relaxing. Massage is a term used to describe a fairly ancient art of healing by touch. It is designed to heal, relieve tension, improve circulation and help the body to rid itself of toxins.

There are different forms of massage. My favourite is massage with aromatherapy oils. There are so many wonderful fragrances to choose from. You can find an aromatherapy masseur locally, but a regular massage will work out quite costly. The best option, if you are both willing, is to take a short course on massage together, buy some gentle oils and massage each other whenever you feel like it. It's also a very sensual activity which will leave your body feeling relaxed and pampered. Make sure you use a very mild oil like lavender. Others may be too strong for during pregnancy, as they can be absorbed through the skin.

DURING PREGNANCY
In the latter stages of pregnancy, when the bones are softening and on the move to prepare for the delivery, you may well feel quite achey some days. Having a loving massage will only help you to feel better physically, but it will also remind you that you are still loved.

Massage is helpful during labour itself, especially if you elect to have a natural delivery. A shoulder and back massage in between contractions works wonders. Even a tummy massage if labour is slow will help you to relax. Alan massaged my face a lot during labour which I found very helpful as I was invariably frowning at the time!

AFTER THE BABY IS BORN

Most of us are not at our best when we have been breast-feeding on 24-hour shifts for many weeks. In those first few weeks of your baby's life you will be working around the clock to provide your baby with all he needs. Your partner's job is to service you, especially if you are breast-feeding which means he can't share the duties in the early weeks. Having a massage after you have put your baby down will help to relax your tense muscles, and also remind you that you have a partner as well as a baby. Babies can be all-consuming initially, and sometimes partners may feel a bit shut out. He will probably welcome the idea of paying some attention to you without the baby in your arms.

You can continue to use massage whenever you both feel the need. I really look forward to mine as it never fails to make me feel as if I've floated off to another planet!

CHAPTER 14

Pregnancy: Common Problems

Pregnancy is a time of great change, particularly in a social and metabolic sense. Sometimes these changes may be accompanied by problems ranging from minor ailments to life-threatening conditions. The quality of your health during pregnancy has a profound influence upon your growing baby, and is influenced by your diet or, more specifically, the balance of individual nutrients. These of course are not the only factors but they are almost certainly the most important which fortunately means that you can do much to help yourself or to prevent or minimise the risk of problems developing. In the ideal situation, a healthy diet and lifestyle during pregnancy is simply an extension of a healthy diet and lifestyle *before* the pregnancy.

EXCESSIVE WEIGHT GAIN

The average weight gain during pregnancy is 12.5 kg (27.6 lb). Some women may gain more. Occasionally there is an increased risk of a mild diabetic state appearing during pregnancy. This would be detected by routine urine tests. Limiting calorie intake, but maintaining a high intake of essential nutrients, including protein, vitamins and minerals, is the best way to limit excess weight gain during pregnancy and reduce the risk of associated diabetes developing. This is particularly important if you are overweight to start with or if you have developed diabetes during a previous pregnancy. In these circumstances women are likely to give birth to babies weighing 4–4.5 kg (9–10 lb) or more. If you have to concentrate on limiting your weight gain, it will be easier in the early stages of pregnancy before nutrient demands increase substantially.

Survey of 448 Mothers
WEIGHT GAIN IN PREGNANCY

The average weight gain in our sample was 12.6 kg (28 lb). 13 women gained 25.2 kg (55½ lb or 4 stone) or more, 5 women gained no weight, and 23 gained less than 3 kg (7 lb or ½ stone).

There was a slightly positive correlation between weight gain in pregnancy and the birth weight of the baby in those women who did not smoke in pregnancy. Most women who were non-smokers and gained more than 14.5 kg (32 lb) were unlikely to give birth to a baby under 2.3 kg (5 lb).

INADEQUATE WEIGHT GAIN

This can be an indicator of inadequate nutrient intake, and can carry with it the risk of poor birth weight for the baby. It appears from recent research that weight gain is less important than the overall nutrient intake and diet quality. Some slim women eat well but have a very active metabolism which means they burn up the extra calories. Conversely, some women of normal weight with reasonable weight gain during pregnancy may in fact be eating poorly which may then jeopardise the growth and development of their baby. Weight changes are routinely measured in ante-natal clinics, though for some women questions about the quality of the diet would be a better way of determining whether nutrient intake is adequate or not.

ANAEMIA

Again it is routine for blood tests to be taken both in the early part and later in the pregnancy to see if anaemia is developing. Haemoglobin falls normally during the course of the pregnancy and may be due to an increased water content of the blood. Iron supplements are often given but usually only when the haemoglobin level has fallen. They are always given with folic acid as this is essential, not only for the development of the baby, but also for forming new red blood cells. Iron supplements should never be taken with tea, coffee or red grape juice as the content of tannin greatly inhibits absorption of this mineral. Taking fruit or fruit juice is ideal as the Vitamin C enhances iron absorption. It is the unabsorbed iron that is the main factor causing digestive symptoms, such as diarrhoea or constipation, which some women experience when taking this supplement.

LOW BIRTH WEIGHT

This is a complex problem. It can potentially be affected by maternal diet but also is greatly influenced by the growth and development of the placenta itself. The quality of maternal blood vessels in the placenta greatly influences the quality of nutrients supplied to the baby. The baby's blood circulation contains levels of many vitamins and minerals that are several times higher than those found in the mother's blood circulation.

157

Some researchers have found that there are increased levels of lead and cadmium in placentas of women who give birth to lower birth-weight babies. Increased placental levels of calcium, iron and zinc have been found in some studies, but not all, to relate to increased birth weights. Some associations have also been made in a large study of 513 women in London between their nutrient intakes in the early stages of pregnancy and the baby's dimensions at birth. Maternal intake of Vitamin B, magnesium, iron and, to a lesser degree, zinc, does seem to be related to the baby's birth weight, head circumference and length. High intakes are associated with greater size, whilst poor intakes are associated with smaller sized babies, especially in those who are of low birth weight. Unfortunately, food and nutritional supplements during the later stages of pregnancy appear to have little effect on reducing the chances of a low birth weight infant.

One British study showed no benefit of zinc supplementation on reducing low birth weight. It is probable that nutritional intake before pregnancy and in the very early stages of pregnancy before attendance at an ante-natal clinic is the crucial factor in determining future growth and development.

There is no disagreement about the important adverse effect of smoking and alcohol on birth weight. It is never too late to stop or reduce consumption of these.

MORNING SICKNESS

This is an all too common problem that affects up to 70 per cent of women at some stage, usually in the early part of their pregnancy. For those who are mildly affected, it normally settles spontaneously by the third or fourth month. If vomiting occurs with weight loss or reduced calorie intake, then nutritional deficiencies can develop. Prolonged severe vomiting can cause profound Vitamin B1 deficiency and disturbance in metabolism. This, in turn, leads to a loss of appetite, delayed emptying of the stomach, and fatigue. Brain damage in the mother has been known to occur as a result of Vitamin B1 deficiency caused by severe morning sickness. Consequently, any woman with more than mild morning sickness, particularly if there is weight loss, should probably take a supplement of Vitamin B complex providing at least 5 mg of Vitamin B1 (thiamin), daily as well as some of the other B vitamins, B2, B3, B6 and B12. Hopefully all women are already taking folic acid.

Morning sickness has also been shown recently to respond to treatment with steroids but these powerful drugs should only be reserved for very severely affected women.

Acupressure, that is pressure on the acupuncture point known as P6, can also help. Commercially available wrist bands that apply pressure at the P6 point are available. This may be a useful first step. You could have a go at acupressure yourself by gently pressing on the P6 point, which is approximately 5 cm (2 inches) above the inner wrist crease, between the two prominent tendons of the lower arm.

Eating 'through' the sickness is important, even if it is liquidised food or fruit milk shakes. Dry crackers often help mild sickness to pass. Eating little and often, taking frequent sips of water and avoiding fatty foods may all be helpful. High-dose Vitamin B6, which has been used in the past, is not of established value and probably should be avoided.

Herbal teas and preparations containing ginger may also have mild anti-nausea effects and are worth trying.

High Blood Pressure

Blood pressure is also measured routinely during pregnancy. Some women have high blood pressure before they are pregnant. Occasionally it may fall due to the opening up of blood vessels during pregnancy. An increase in blood pressure during the early stages of pregnancy is an important warning sign and treatment may be required. Unchecked, it may develop into pre-eclampsia (see below).

PRE-ECLAMPSIA

Pre-eclampsia is a condition related to the health and activity of the placenta. Increasing blood pressure, disturbances in kidney and liver function, fluid retention and protein in the urine are features. Pre-eclampsia typically, if untreated, will lead on to the development of eclampsia – severe epileptic fits, accompanied by a very high blood pressure. This is a disastrous event with serious increased risk of death for the mother and baby alike.

The cause of pre-eclampsia is uncertain. It is more likely to occur in women who are severely obese or who have experienced pre-eclampsia in a previous pregnancy. The presence of any protein in the urine suggests the development of pre-eclampsia, although it can be due to urine infection or kidney problems. Doctors need to be on the lookout for the early signs of pre-eclampsia which is still often missed or detected late in the pregnancy.

Pre-eclampsia is normally treated by rest and drugs to control the blood pressure. Salt restriction is not advisable during pregnancy as it is known to be dangerous. Increased calcium intake in the diet might be helpful and large studies in the United States are under way currently to assess this. Magnesium, given usually by injections, is a popular treatment in the United States for controlling blood pressure in pre-eclampsia and in developed eclampsia. However, it is rarely used in the United Kingdom. Its exact value will be determined by future studies being conducted in South Africa. Magnesium supplements in tablet form have been given safely during pregnancy, and might prove to be a useful alternative.

Risk of pre-eclampsia might be related to a number of, as yet, unknown unidentified nutritional factors, including overall nutrient intake (see below).

ECLAMPSIA

Eclampsia consists of epileptic-like convulsions in association with pre-eclampsia. However, high blood pressure, fluid retention or protein in the urine may not always be present as warning signs before the development of eclampsia. Eclampsia occurs in one in 2,000 pregnancies in the United Kingdom. Two per cent of such women die and 35 per cent have experienced major ill-health as a result. Of the babies 2 per cent are still-born, and 3.5 per cent die shortly after birth. Eclampsia can occur shortly after birth as well as before or during labour itself. Pregnant teenagers, many of whom have poor nutrient intakes, are apparently three times more likely than older women to have eclamptic fits. Careful monitoring in the ante-natal clinic is vital, and warning symptoms such as headache, visual disturbance and indigestion should be taken seriously.

JAUNDICE DURING PREGNANCY

Occasionally jaundice develops during pregnancy. Disturbances in liver function result in the accumulation of the yellow pigment, bile, in the bloodstream. Occasionally this runs in the family or there may be a history of jaundice occurring when on the oral contraceptive pill. Specialist treatment is required. Supplements of Vitamin K and other nutrients may also be required. The first symptom of this liver problem in pregnancy may be increased skin itching or dark discoloration of urine.

CONSTIPATION AND PILES

Occasionally constipation develops during pregnancy. Ensuring a good intake of fibre, especially from fruit and vegetables, supplements of some seeds, including sunflower seeds and linseeds, and use of mild laxatives, especially magnesium in tablet or liquid form, will usually correct the problems. Try not to use bran. Ordinary coarse oats, porridge or muesli are a better bet.

Continuing constipation, especially towards the end of pregnancy, can contribute to the development of haemorrhoids or piles. These, in part, are due to the greatly increased blood supply in the pelvis, together with the down-bearing pressure of the ever-expanding uterus and baby. Putting your feet up, even lying on the floor with them elevated against a wall, can help reduce the swelling and discomfort from piles. If you develop haemorrhoids you may also need to use some strong ointment or herbal cream.

HEARTBURN

Space within the abdomen is at a premium during pregnancy, and pressure on the stomach means that some of the acid is pushed up into the lower end of the oesophagus or gullet, producing discomfort and heartburn. This is more likely to occur towards the end of pregnancy, especially when bending or lying. Sitting upright after meals, using more pillows in bed, or raising the head of the bed may help. Anti-acid preparations of magnesium combined with a gelatinous agent to reduce the ease with which acid washes back into the gullet are helpful and safe agents to use. Ask your doctor or pharmacist.

MUSCLE CRAMPS

These are particularly likely to occur towards the end of pregnancy, perhaps because baby is taking so many of the minerals, including calcium, magnesium, potassium and sodium. Again, ensuring a good diet is important. Taking extra sodium (salt) is unwise, but ensuring a good supply of calcium, magnesium and potassium in the diet is important. Eating plenty of dairy products for calcium, fruit and vegetables for magnesium, and nuts and seeds may help.

BACKACHE

This is a common problem and can be influenced by underlying spinal or muscle problems, injury (recent or in the past), together with the hormonal changes of pregnancy. A hormone, relaxin, softens connective tissues around the pelvis towards the end of pregnancy and this can aggravate back and other aches and pains. If severe, rest is essential, and a visit to an osteopath may be beneficial. Gentle treatment is likely to ease your back into alignment and comfort as a result. Heat, massage and swimming may all be helpful.

SKIN PIGMENTATION

Increased darkening of the skin occurs due to the change in hormones. Sometimes skin pigmentation can develop on

163

the face (chloasma). This is part of the hormonal changes of pregnancy and usually resolves after delivery. Women often notice they tan quickly when exposed to even small amounts of sunlight while they are pregnant.

HEARING LOSS

Occasionally hearing loss develops from pregnancy, which always requires a medical check-up. It is probably due to wax in the ears and sometimes it is due to a particular sensitivity to the hormone, oestrogen. If this latter is the cause, then women who suffer with loss of hearing during pregnancy must not take the oral contraceptive pill or HRT in later life.

CARPAL TUNNEL SYNDROME

A tingling in the hands and fingers can be due to compression on a nerve at the wrist due to fluid retention and weight gain. Wearing wrist splints at night may be helpful, and preventing excessive weight gain may be important. Supplements of high doses of Vitamin B have been tried in non-pregnant women but this is not advisable during pregnancy.

PART THREE
Healthy Baby

CHAPTER 15

Feeding Your Baby

Once you discover that you are pregnant, the emphasis for the first nine months probably centres on growing a healthy baby and surviving the delivery. The chat is very much about your changing shape, your appetite, changing energy levels and the choices of the inevitable labour. During the latter stages of pregnancy we prepare the nursery (or in our case, the corner of our room, as we always had our babies with us for the first few months), and gather a collection of tiny, cute unisex clothes. The ante-natal classes focus on our labour choices and we touch on the subject of feeding the baby, in particular the benefits of breast-feeding. And that in my experience is usually where it ends. We are then left to work the rest out for ourselves.

When we did our first ante-natal classes some fifteen years ago, the National Childbirth Trust (NCT) conveyed the benefits of breast-feeding in no uncertain terms. If there was ever any doubt in my mind, which there wasn't because I honestly had never really thought about it, it was soon dissipated. I rushed out and bought the fattest book on the subject called *Everything You Wanted to Know about Breast-Feeding and Were Too Afraid to Ask*, which unbeknownst to me at the time would get me out of more than one corner in the years to come. Sadly this book is no longer in print, but looking back I don't know what I would have done without it.

Even to this day, despite the fact that there are a variety of classes covering the choices we have in labour, there are still grossly inadequate facilities to teach new mums how to go about feeding their infants, and indeed how to wean them when the time comes. Considering the vital importance of good nutrition up to and including the first precious year of life it seems a little ludicrous, doesn't it?

With four children and a busy advisory service to run, I have not had the time to even encourage others to set up courses around the country. However, this book will give you much of the vital information that you need, and if we all make a little time we could successfully campaign for changes.

Survey of 448 Mothers
BREAST-FEEDING HABITS

---

307 (68%) of the women in our survey breast-fed their first child. Of the remaining 32%, only 11 went on to breast-feed their second child.

BREAST IS BEST

Breast is Best is not only the title of a wonderful book by Doctors Penny and Andrew Stanway, but it is also the message that the World Health Organisation actively works to convey. All mammals produce tailor-made milk for their young, and woman is no exception. Mother Nature, in her usual amazing style, ensures that breast-milk provides all the vital nutrients that a growing baby needs, as well as supplying them with immunity to infectious diseases and resistance to germs around them. The natural immunity which is passed from mothers to their breast-fed children stays with them, not only during infanthood, but into their young childhood.

Breast-milk contains protein, fat, sugar, amino acids, enzymes, vitamins, minerals and trace elements. Some of the fats are specialised, long-chain polyunsaturated fatty acids, also known as essential fatty acids, which are necessary for the developing brain and retina (the light-sensitive part of the eye). The baby's brain grows rapidly during the last three months of pregnancy and during the first year after birth. At this time it accounts for some 10 per cent of total body weight, and demands 60 per cent of the baby's total energy intake! As babies cannot easily convert these long-chain polyunsaturated fatty acids, they rely on a supply from the mother across the placenta during pregnancy and from the breast-milk after birth. As yet formula milk in the UK does not contain these specialised fats, but some manufacturers are considering adding evening primrose oil and marine oils to infant milks, especially those for premature babies.

ADVANTAGES FOR MUM

★ **It's all done for you** Once breast-feeding is established, the amount of milk you produce is decided by your baby. It is a system of supply and demand. The length of time and frequency of your baby's feeds will determine how much milk is required.

★ **Less expense and bother** You will not need to continually pay for milk powder nor have the expense of sterilising equipment or feeding bottles. Neither will you need to carry supplies of milk in your bag when you go out.

★ **More convenient** There is no warming of bottles as breast-milk is always the right temperature for your baby.

You will certainly be glad you chose to breast-feed in the middle of the night; so too will your partner if you share duties!

★ **More peaceful**   Breast-feeding is both very relaxing and sensual. It brings mothers naturally closer to their offspring, which is calming to the baby. In fact research shows that breast-fed babies cry less than those bottle-fed, probably because they feel more secure.

★ **More healthy**   Mother Nature intended us to breast-feed our young for good reason. Women who breast-feed their children for long periods actually have a lower rate of breast cancer than women who never breast-fed.

★ **More intelligent children**   Both American and British studies have shown that there is a significant developmental difference in breast-fed babies, and that their performance in vocabulary and hand-eye co-ordination tests is better than bottle-fed children. Doing the best for your baby pays dividends that both you and your partner can enjoy later on.

★ **Less smelly nappies**   Because breast-milk is much easier to digest than synthetic feeds, there is much less waste, and what is left doesn't smell unpleasant, which has to be an added bonus!

★ **No periods for longer**   When you are fully breast-feeding, your body knows that you are not ready to conceive again. Ovulation is suspended and so too are your monthly periods. Some women remain period-free for in excess of six months after giving birth, which gives their iron stores a chance to build up at a time when the growing baby's iron stores are running low.

★ **Contraceptive value**   Whilst you are fully breast-feeding during the first few months of your baby's life, and not ovulating, you probably will not need to use contraceptives. However, as breast-feeding in later months is not 100 per cent protective, it is advisable to use other precautions, preferably other than the contraceptive pill.

★ **Far more fulfilling** The whole experience of having the baby on your breast, next to your skin, and the fact that your body continues to provide a lifeline to the baby, just as it did during pregnancy, is wondrous. It is a very moving and satisfying experience, which in my opinion, no woman who is able to breast-feed should deny herself.

ADVANTAGES FOR BABY

★ **Provides security** Breast-feeding, or nursing as it is otherwise known, allows the baby close contact with her mother's warm skin, where the heartbeat that she has grown so used to hearing can still be heard.

★ **More comfort** At feeding time the baby still feels as if she is part of the environment that she has been used to during her growing phase in the womb. The contact the baby experiences at feeding time allows her to explore her mother's physical features at close range whilst enjoying being stroked and cuddled.

★ **Increased tranquillity** Research shows that breast-fed babies are likely to be more content with their lot, less afraid, less jealous and not so spiteful as their bottle-fed counterparts.

★ **Less tummy upset** A breast-fed baby is less likely to become constipated or to suffer with colic than those who are given substitutes. As breast-milk is tailor-made for your baby, it follows that it is more easily digested.

★ **Fewer health problems** Breast-feeding encourages the growth in the baby's gut of millions of healthy bacteria which help to dispel those that can cause diarrhoea. A breast-fed baby is less likely to succumb to gastroenteritis or chest infections, and is much less likely to contract allergies and coeliac disease (gluten intolerance) in later life. This is particularly important if there is a family history of allergy.

171

★ **Less likely to be fat** Because the fats in breast-milk are different from the fats found in formula milk, the breast-fed baby has a considerably reduced chance of becoming a fat adult. As fat adults are more prone to heart disease, high levels of cholesterol, high blood pressure and diabetes, you will be giving your baby the best possible chance of good health if you do decide to breast-feed.

THE BEST ALL-ROUND OPTION

Not only is breast-feeding better for both mothers and babies, it is also a way of conserving world resources. With world population on the increase, bottle-fed babies will be making even greater demands on cows who will need even more space to graze, which results in the destruction of even more forestland. There is also the extra transportation involved in delivering cow's milk, the energy it takes to convert the milk into formula, and the waste products that result from the milk (the tins, for instance, which are rarely recycled). Neither does this take into account the manufacture of bottles, teats and sterilising equipment . . .

The wonders of Mother Nature never cease to amaze me. The whole process of making and growing a baby is a near miracle, and on top of that we are provided with breast-milk, the most perfect food for our growing child. By breast-feeding you will be able to continue to provide all the nutrients that your baby needs for the first four months of life, just as you did via the placenta when the baby was growing inside your body. Despite some initial problems which some women experience when breast-feeding, once the routine is established it is an indescribable joy to nurse a baby, and one of the most fulfilling bonuses of mothering.

Survey of 448 Mothers
BREAST-FEEDING DURATION

---

308 women had only one child, 210 of whom breast-fed.
Of the 140 women (31.2%) who went on to have more than one child, 91 women breast-fed for an average of 16.2 weeks.

WHO CAN'T BREAST-FEED?

I always ask patients whether they breast-fed their children. All too often I am told that they began for a few days or weeks, and then were advised to give up as 'they didn't have enough milk'. This is often a fallacy. Breast-feeding is all about supply and demand. If you continue to feed your baby on demand, in other words when the baby calls out for a feed, your breasts will be stimulated to produce sufficient milk to meet your baby's demand.

Unless you became very sick, your milk supply would remain unaffected. I have even continued to feed two of my babies through horrendous breast infections with a fever of 104°F! So if breast-milk is such a perfect and constant supply of nutrients, why is it that so many women choose to bottle-feed initially, or end up bottle-feeding for longer than six weeks? In the UK an average 64 per cent of babies begin life being breast-fed, but by six weeks only three in five are still being put to the breast, despite the fact that the majority of women questioned would have preferred to continue feeding. As recently as fifty years ago, nine out of ten babies were breast-fed, many of them for more than six months.

Research shows that poor professional advice is the reason why so many women give up feeding or don't even seriously consider the option in the first place. Women are given incorrect or inadequate advice about overcoming the problems that often arise, and bow to the better judgement of the health adviser who 'obviously knows best'. For example, a falling milk supply can be remedied by feeding more often, or using a breast pump to stimulate milk production. If I had a pound for every health visitor who told mums with milk-flow problems to substitute with formula, or to give other drinks to the baby in between feeds, especially in the summer, I would no longer need to buy my weekly lottery ticket! When you consider that the health of all future generations depends on this advice, it shows that there is a very real need for improved training for our health-care professionals.

The social pressures faced by women who opt to breast-feed are great enough without being fed false information. Anyone who has breast-fed for any length of time will tell you what a performance it is being out shopping with a breast-fed baby at feed-time. There are so few shops that provide nursing facilities, and our society still does not expect to see mums feeding their babies in public places. When we return to work there is little flexibility to help us continue feeding, and the aggressive marketing by the milk formula manufacturers makes it all too easy for a struggling mother to succumb.

So whilst we wait for governments to intervene and health-care professionals to become better trained, it's down to you to weigh up the pros and cons of breast-feeding. If you cannot breast-feed your baby for whatever reason do make sure that you:

★ make up the feeds according to the instructions
★ sterilise the bottles and teats properly
★ test the temperature of a heated feed before offering it to the baby
★ don't use the microwave to heat baby milk as it changes the nutritional composition of the milk, and can give uneven heating

★ discard any milk remaining in the bottle after a feed
★ look at changing the formula you have chosen, if your baby shows signs of discomfort, or allergy symptoms

These instructions should be taken very seriously because it is thought that a staggering one and a half million babies in the world die each year from unhygienic bottle feeding, mainly in the third world. Bottle-fed babies stand nearly double the chance of developing diabetes than those that are breast-fed, and are also at higher risk of developing heart disease later in life. No matter how hard the formula milk manufacturers try, it is impossible to exactly replicate breast-milk. Unless you have no alternative, breast-milk will probably always be the best option.

How To Breast-Feed

Many women naturally go through at least one stage of panic about breast-feeding, wondering whether they will be able to feed and whether they will have enough milk to sustain this new precious little person. Nourishing a baby, without any external help, is an extremely responsible job, and not one that we are given much training for. Surprisingly, once you get started, especially if you have a little knowledge, it is easier than it might appear. Our fellow mammals seem to get it right without going to classes, so it stands to reason that much of the technique should be instinctive.

Whilst some women take to breast-feeding like a duck takes to water, never encountering any problems, others battle on with unforeseen events. Unforeseen because no-one ever told them that there are surmountable pitfalls. In order to remain composed and confident I firmly believe that women should be aware of what could go wrong and how to correct it before the event.

You will need to come to terms with the fact that breast-feeding takes time, especially if you have recently given up a busy demanding job. This is your new job for the next few months, I called it my 'Daisy the Cow Syndrome'! Making a safe, calm environment for both you and your baby, and not worrying about the 'outside world' are high on the agenda for you during those first few weeks. Not so long ago women had a 'lying-in' period, which lasted for about a month after having their babies – that is they were expected to stay in bed for four weeks attending to their baby's needs and resting in between, whilst the rest of the family waited on them. So don't feel guilty if you achieve nothing more than nourishing your baby, eating well, drinking plenty and resting for the first few weeks. Get your partner to ration those well-meaning visitors to certain hours of the day so that you are able to relax.

A FEW BREAST-FEEDING RULES
When you start breast-feeding, there are a few 'rules' that you should try to follow. Your own comfort, and that of the baby, will depend on it.

★ **A quiet, peaceful environment**   You need to feel relaxed and at ease, without any external demands or interruptions, and with no time limit.
★ **A feeding chair or adequate support**   Successful breast-feeding is related to position. In those first days when you are likely to be feeding the baby in bed, make sure that you put a cushion under the baby so that she can roll in your arms to reach your nipple without you having to contort your body.
★ **Feed from both breasts**   Make sure right from the start that your baby feeds from both breasts equally. You have fore-milk, which is more like a drink, and hind-milk to follow, which is her food. It is important to empty both

breasts regularly, otherwise you are likely to get engorged, with hard, red, painful, lumpy breasts! If your baby has had enough after the first breast, remember to offer her the full second breast at the next feed.

★ **Drink plenty**   Have a large mug of decaffeinated or herbal tea, water or fruit juice by you, so that you can replenish your stocks during the feed. When I first started feeding, Alan brought home a pint mug as a joke, but it actually got used at every feed as I was so thirsty.

★ **Get fitted for your feeding bras**   Many breast problems occur because of ill-fitting feeding bras. It is vital that you wear a comfortable feeding bra that does not restrict your milk supply. In the early days, when your breasts are acclimatising themselves to your baby's needs, you may need to wear a night-time bra also. The NCT have breast-feeding counsellors who will fit you, as do good department stores.

★ **Keep your nipples clean and dry**   Splash your nipples with water and pat them dry. Don't use soap or cleansing gel whilst you are feeding.

★ **Feed on demand**   Breast-feeding, unlike bottle-feeding, is meant to be performed on demand. Breast-milk quality and concentration varies during the day according to your baby's needs, unlike formula milk, which is the same at every feed. Your baby may need feeding every few hours for some weeks and should be put to the breast whenever she wakes with a hunger cry, which you will come to recognise. Breast-fed babies sleep less than those on the bottle, so don't be persuaded that you are not satisfying your breast-fed baby because she asks for more feeds. She is simply demanding good nutrients at the rate at which she can digest them. Unless she stops growing, you need not have any cause for concern.

★ **Resist the temptation to use a dummy**   When babies spend hours sucking on a dummy they are less likely to be able to stimulate your breasts to produce adequate milk. So the few hours' peace and quiet you get from the dummy will be cancelled out by the frustration you will no doubt encounter later when you have milk-supply problems, and as a result an unhappy and unsatisfied baby.

★ **Rest with your baby**   As you will be doing the night shift as well as the day shift, you will need to rest with your baby. As the baby develops its own little pattern, you will know when you have a few hours to get your head down. If you get overtired you will feel awful and you will not be an efficient 'cow'!

★ **Don't listen to old wives' tales**   When you have just given birth you will find that well-meaning friends and relatives crawl out of the woodwork to give you advice. They may tell you that giving the odd bottle of formula will help the baby to grow, or that breast-fed babies need extra fluid, or that your milk looks too thin, or the way to prevent sore nipples is to feed every four hours.

COMMON PROBLEMS WITH BREAST-FEEDING

If you are a first-time mother then it may be particularly useful to know how to deal with some of these problems. Most of them respond to early and prompt treatment without disturbing the breast-feeding process.

ENGORGED BREASTS
For the first few days after giving birth your breasts will supply colostrum to your baby. This is a yellow fluid designed to get your baby's digestive system going, and contains all the protein, fats, vitamins and minerals that your baby needs. It is also a concentrated source of antibodies which give your baby protection against infection.

On about the third day the actual milk arrives and by the fifth day you may well feel that you have more milk than United Dairies. Until your breasts and your baby have sorted what is actually required, it is likely that you may suddenly find you wake up with rock-hard, painful, lumpy bosoms. Don't despair, get in the bath and massage your breasts with a warm flannel. Gently express some of the excess milk and then feed your baby. This should all settle down within a few days.

SORE NIPPLES

As your nipples are only used to being fondled during love-making, it is likely that they may get sore initially as a baby's suction is quite strong. There are several ways of coping.

★ Make sure you position the baby correctly on the breast so that your whole nipple is in her mouth. Support her with pillows as necessary.

★ Don't pull the baby off the breast, but instead place your little finger gently in the corner of her mouth to break the suction.

★ Put a little breast-milk on your nipples after a feed and leave them to dry naturally.

★ Use a healing cream in between feeds, like Camillosan.

★ Avoid using plastic-backed breast pads as they cause your nipples to sweat and prolong the soreness.

★ If possible expose your nipples to sunlight for short regular periods.

★ Wear cotton feeding bras instead of man-made fibres as they will allow air to circulate freely.

★ Feed from the least sore side first.

★ If your nipples become really cracked get some advice about nipple shields which can be used in the short term whilst your nipples are healing.

MASTITIS

Whilst breast-feeding women sometimes get inflammation of the breast tissue, or mastitis, as a result of a blocked milk duct in the breast which can then lead to infection. Mastitis can usually be handled by regular massage of the breast with hot flannels and by expressing milk between feeds, either by hand or with a pump. Antibiotics may be needed if a fever develops. It is a painful experience, but a condition that passes relatively quickly.

BREAST ABSCESS

This unfortunate problem causes a painful breast lump, accompanied by high fever, and needs to be dealt with very quickly by your doctor. You will often need to take a course of antibiotics. The most sensible thing to do is to continue to feed through it despite the pain. The alternative is to stop feeding your baby, at which time your breasts are likely to become engorged and feel even more painful. I managed to feed through several breast abscesses which occurred when my babies were several months old. Although it made me grit my teeth at the time, I was so glad that I had persevered afterwards, as I was able to continue to breast-feed.

'INSUFFICIENT MILK'

If you feel that your milk supply is dwindling you will need to put your baby to the breast more often. It takes about forty-eight hours to increase your milk supply, so be patient. Unless you are taking any medication which is likely to interfere with your breast-milk, and you are eating well and drinking plenty, there is no reason why your milk supply won't build up.

FEEDING IN PUBLIC

It is quite normal to feel self-conscious about exposing your breasts in public, especially in front of people you know, like great-uncles! People won't be offended if you ask to use a separate room, especially during the first few weeks when your self-consciousness is likely to be at its height, whilst you are lacking confidence in your feeding technique. The other way around the problem is to wear T-shirts, sweat-shirts or loose-fitting jumpers which you can raise to the appropriate level without showing much at all. If you carry a muslin nappy with you as a feeding cloth, if any bits do show you can cover them up quite easily.

FEEDING AND WORKING

If you only have six weeks' maternity leave, you might be tempted to switch your baby to formula milk unless you are very determined. Expressing milk is not particularly difficult when you get the hang of it, it just takes a little while to settle on a method that suits you. You have several options: hand pumping, which I found very slow; a manual breast pump, which is inexpensive and very efficient once you get going; or you can hire an electric pump, which will also do the job efficiently.

It is best to wait until your feeding is really established before pumping milk off, probably at least four weeks. Then you can pump away in between feeds and freeze the milk in little polythene bags, like the Playtex bags, for example. Playtex bottles and teats are usually accepted by breast-fed babies. Your carer simply defrosts the milk in your absence and inserts it into the Playtex bottle, without it being touched by human hands.

If you decide to use a manual pump, you can take the pump to work with you and express milk at feed times. I would recommend going back to work part-time if at all possible, and if you live close enough, asking your carer to bring the baby in for a lunch-time feed. You will obviously have to evaluate your own situation, remembering that the future health of your baby is at stake.

You will need to invest in a good book on the subject of breast-feeding. *Breast is Best* is a must, as is *The National Childbirth Trust Book of Pregnancy, Birth and Parenthood*. Further details about these can be found on page 277. But most of all, enjoy every minute of your feeding. It's a precious time that you will look back on with pride for the rest of your life.

CHAPTER 16

Feeding Your Baby: Common Questions Answered

We are so constantly bombarded with conflicting information about how to feed and wean our babies, that you are almost entitled to feel confused. This section concentrates on setting the record straight, according to current research, about common problems you might encounter and questions that are often asked.

Q: *How long is it safe for me to breast-feed my baby?*

A: Both the World Health Organisation and the Department of Health in their recent report, 'Weaning and the Weaning Diet', consider that breast-milk supplies the baby with all the nutrients needed until it reaches the age of four months. At about four months we need to start introducing solid food as well as continuing to breast-feed the baby. There is no precise time to give up feeding, though. Babies will often indicate to us when they have had enough. The quality of breast-milk declines after six months, but together with solid foods, and vitamin drops, you can continue to breast-feed for as long as both you and your baby are happy to do so. The vast majority of women stop breast-feeding within the first year, but some women do go on feeding until their children are two or three.

Q: *My baby doesn't seem to be interested in food. He is five months old but isn't showing any signs of wanting to feed. I feel frustrated and wonder whether my milk is providing him with all he needs?*

A: Healthy babies tend to start on solids when they are ready, provided you give them a taste that they like. It is possible that you haven't hit on a tempting flavour to start, so you may just need to experiment more, until you find something that he will take to. If he is growing steadily, you need not be too concerned for the next month or so. You will soon need to give him some multi-vitamin drops and some iron, as the levels in your breast-milk at this stage are likely to be less adequate. I would suggest that you make an appointment with your health visitor to discuss the problem and ask her to supply the vitamin and mineral supplements.

Q: *What about alcohol during breast feeding?*

A: Although alcohol does get into the breast-milk, the toxic component, aldehydes, do not get through the breast to the baby. Whilst some babies seem to tolerate an occasional drink, others seem to develop colic and irritability. If your baby seems to cope then there is no harm in enjoying the occasional drink.

   If you drink enough alcohol to alter your mood, it may well interfere with the let-down reflex when you are breast-feeding. Alcohol inhibits the production of the hormone oxytocin, which is responsible for letting the milk flow out the milk ducts into the breast. So as well as too much alcohol being bad for your baby, it is likely to hinder the natural breast-feeding mechanism.

184

Q: *Does smoking affect the quality of breast-milk?*

A: Smoking before a breast-feed can result in higher levels of nicotine in your breast-milk than in your blood. Babies of heavy smokers are likely to feel sick and restless as a result of the amount of nicotine that they receive through the breast-milk. And, as with alcohol, the effect of nicotine being released into your bloodstream can affect the let-down mechanism of your milk supply. Don't forget about the dangers of passive smoking either.

Q: *What should I do about medical drugs whilst breast-feeding?*

A: Do not take any drug, high-dose nutritional supplement, herbal preparation or over-the-counter preparation, without checking first with your doctor or pharmacist. Unqualified advice from friends and relatives, no matter how well-meaning, or from unqualified shop assistants, is no substitute.

An important difference when breast-feeding is that your baby could be allergic to a drug that you are taking, even though you are not. This is rare, but possible.

A number of drugs may interfere with milk supply, including steroids and diuretics. Antibiotics, if taken, can pass to the baby and, as a side-effect, can induce diarrhoea. This is usually self-limiting, but they might precipitate an episode of thrush in your baby that could require treatment with creams or medicine by mouth. Anti-depressant drugs are sometimes needed in those who suffer from post-natal depression. Some can safely be used whilst breast-feeding, but again, expert advice is required. Sedative drugs should be avoided wherever possible. They pass into the breast-milk and will sedate the baby, sometimes to a point that will reduce its natural wakefulness and feeding instincts.

Laxatives – again many of the more powerful laxatives, including senna, herbal preparations and some drugs – will pass into the breast-milk, giving your baby an unneeded dose.

If it is necessary for you to take a drug on an intermittent basis, such as a painkiller, then try to take this away from the time when you will be feeding. Blood levels normally reach their peak within one or two hours of taking a tablet, and concentration in the breast-milk will rise after this time too. For example, if there is a gap of several hours when you will not be breast-feeding, such as at night, then this might be a better time to take the drug than during the day.

Q: *I have heard that it is not advisable to breast-feed a baby after the age of six months because of the declining quality of my milk. Is this true?*

A: The quality of your breast-milk does deteriorate after six months, for example it will not contain sufficient iron to satisfy your baby's requirements, and zinc and copper are likely to be in short supply. However, you will be introducing your baby to solids at four months, and concentrating on foods that are rich in nutrients, in order to make up the short-fall. As long as you are eating well and your baby gets plenty of daylight, and has fruit and vegetables at each meal, you will be doing well. The Department of Health do recommend that breast-fed babies over the age of six months have supplements of Vitamins A and D. You can buy these in any chemist or get them from your health visitor.

Q: *My mother commented that my milk looks thin, and I wonder how to tell whether it is of sufficient quality to fulfil my baby's needs?*

A: The texture of breast-milk tends to vary at different times of the day. You also need to remember that you have both fore-milk, which is a thin liquid designed as a drink, and the denser hind-milk which is regarded as the food. If your baby is still gaining weight and you are eating a healthy diet, I don't think you have any cause for concern.

Q: *How can you tell whether your baby is getting enough milk from the breast?*

A: If your baby is growing steadily, seems contented and is producing wet nappies, you can assume that she is getting enough milk. If you want to build up your milk supply further, you will need to put her to your breast more frequently, and make sure that she empties each breast before swapping her over.

Q: *My baby is six months old and has been happily breast-feeding since birth. Recently he has started to turn his head away from my breast, and I have to coax him to feed. Is he trying to tell me he has had enough breast-milk?*

A: Some babies do give up breast-feeding of their own accord, but with such a young baby, who was feeding happily, it is more likely that there is some other problem that needs to be addressed. Perhaps he is teething, and therefore finding feeding uncomfortable. Try using some Chamomilla homoeopathic teething granules, or rub some Bonjela on to his gums a little while before a feed. Alternatively, you should review your diet to see whether something you have eaten has put him off! Breast-milk can take on the flavour of the food you eat. If neither of those solutions help, I would suggest contacting a breast-feeding counsellor. You will find some useful telephone numbers on page 279.

Q: *I have read that even breast-fed babies should be given vitamin supplements from the age of one month, is this really true?*

A: Current guidelines laid down by the Department of Health state that babies who are being breast-fed, who are thought likely to have good vitamin stores because the mother had a good diet leading up to and during pregnancy, should not need to take vitamin supplements until the age of six months. Where there is any doubt about the nutritional status of the mother, it is advised that supplementation begin at one month. At six months babies should be given supplements, which they should continue until they are at least five years of age.

Q: *My baby is only five and a half months, but guzzles everything I offer her and still appears to want more. She is still fully breast-fed plus has three baby meals per day. Should I go along with her demands or restrict her intake of solids as she is so young?*

A: Unless your baby is gaining too much weight there is no reason why you can't be guided by her apparent needs. As long as she continues to breast-feed well and you offer her foods that are suitable for her age, including finger foods (see page 200), you should not run into any problems. She may be having a growth spurt, which would account for her healthy appetite.

Q: *I have offered my nine-month-old baby all the suitable vegetables, but cannot interest him in any of them. Am I right in assuming that he will be lacking in vitamins and minerals as a result?*

A: Vegetables are a very important part of your baby's diet as they contain lots of Vitamin C and fibre, but some babies simply refuse them. Try making some vegetable soups or mixing small pieces of vegetables with mince to disguise them. Sometimes babies prefer sweet flavours, and as breast-milk tends to be sweet you can try mixing this with puréed vegetables. Carrots and sweet potatoes have a sweet flavour, so try those first.

Q: *Our daughter has just cut her first two teeth and my family are joking about her biting my nipples. Is she likely to?*

A: Most babies don't use their teeth to feed, and they don't make a habit of biting, except in play or by accident. If your baby does start to bite, tell her firmly not to and she will eventually get the message. Women have fed children with a full set of teeth and still come out with two nipples intact!

Q: *I have been giving our little boy a main course and a dessert for the last few weeks at each meal-time. Now he has started to refuse the savoury course, no matter how I try to tempt him, and won't eat until I give him the chocolate pudding or peach custard first. How can I re-interest him in wholesome food?*

A: It seems that your baby not only knows what he likes, but is also trying to lay down the law. Whilst those artificially sweet foods are very palatable, they will not deliver the goods in terms of nutrients. I suggest you show who is boss, and offer only savoury food, until the message gets through. After a few tantrums, he will probably forget about chocolate pudding, at which point you can introduce stewed fresh or dried fruit, which is intrinsically sweet, and much more nutritious.

Q: *I weaned our daughter from the breast at four months because of returning to work. She has been having bottles of formula milk instead. She is now thirteen months, and I can't get her to give up her night-time bottles. Will she give up naturally at some point?*

A: She is probably clinging on to her bottle for comfort. Give her a feeder cup instead, as an interim measure, so that she still has the drink without the bottle. If she is disturbed in the night, go in and give her some reassurance and tuck her in. After a while she will forget about the night-time bottle, and lose interest in the drink in the cup until the morning.

Q: *We are vegetarians and I want to start introducing solids to our son who is four months old. When can I start to give him vegetarian proteins like peas and beans?*

A: You can introduce small amounts of these between four and six months, preferably mixed with some breast- or formula milk. Beans are more difficult to digest, so should not be included in your baby's diet until he is six or seven months. Many vegetarian foods contain high levels of phytic acid which tends to inhibit the absorption particularly of iron, zinc and calcium. Foods to watch out for are wholewheat cereal and bran products. Having foods which are rich in Vitamin C with each meal will help, and giving a multi-vitamin and multi-mineral preparation will do the rest.

Q: *My husband has an allergy to cow's milk and I am unable to tolerate wheat. How can we tell whether our new baby is likely to have similar allergies, and what should we do about it if she has?*

A: In view of your family history, you should err on the side of caution. Wait until your baby is nine months of age before introducing either groups of foods. Then introduce small amounts of dairy products, like yoghurt, cheese and whole cow's milk to mix with solids, and watch for a reaction for a few weeks before taking any further action, If after careful consideration your baby seems fine with dairy products, then move on to small amounts of wheat and repeat the exercise. The longer you leave it to try, the less chance there will be of an adverse reaction. Many children have transient sensitivities that they grow out of as they grow older. If you have concerns, then make an appointment to see your doctor.

Q: *Our baby is eleven months now, but still has his bottle of milk in the night. We have tried to get him to do without, but he wakes up and won't settle until we give in. He appears to be hungry, do you think I should feed him more during the day?*

A: It is possible that your baby cannot last from sunset to sunrise without some food, especially if he goes to bed early in the evening. However, the bottle in the night may just be habit, or comfort. Make sure he has a hearty evening meal and milk-feed, and perhaps offer him more to eat at other meals. Substitute the night-time bottle for a feeding cup, still containing milk, and show him where to find the cup in case he is hungry. If the cup is emptied on a regular basis you know that he is hungry. However, if he forgets about the cup, you will have just broken a

191

habit that would have needed to be dealt with sooner or later.

Q: *I am fully breast-feeding our baby who is now three months old. So far we have not been using contraception as we were told that we wouldn't need to until I started mixed feeding. I have since been told that this is not true. I don't want another baby yet, and I am feeling a bit confused.*

A: Breast-feeding suppresses ovulation and usually you remain period-free. Initially, if you are fully breast-feeding you will probably be protected, but the trouble is it is unlikely that you will know when your fertility returns. For that reason, after the first few months it is wise to take other contraceptive precautions.

Q: *My husband is keen to help me with our new baby, but because I'm breast-feeding, how can he be of help? Have you any suggestions?*

A: Yes, many, having been there myself. Although he can't feed the baby for you initially, once your feeding is established, you can pump off enough milk during the day so that your partner can do at least one night feed, giving you a bigger stretch of sleep. That will make a lot of difference. He can also help with the housework, prepare meals for you and give you a regular massage and lots of reassurance. You will feel better for having extra sleep, and he will feel satisfied that he is contributing.

Q: *My husband has brought a dummy for me to give the baby as she has been ratty and unsettled recently. She seems to like it, but I have heard conflicting reports about dummies. Will I spoil her teeth?*

A: Whilst dummies, or pacifiers as they are sometimes known, often solve the short-term problem, they can cause others. For example, after sucking a dummy for hours your baby will be less likely to want to suck on your breast to stimulate the milk supply. Also dummies, if used regularly, can alter the shape of the jaw, which may present dental and speech problems later on. Occasional use is probably fine, but try not to get your baby attached to a dummy. Your clean little finger might be used as a dummy on the odd occasion.

Both your health visitor and the National Childbirth Trust will be happy to give you further advice. Don't be afraid to ask!

CHAPTER 17

Weaning Stage One:
From Four to Six Months

There are no hard and fast rules about when exactly to introduce your baby to real food, otherwise known as solids, (although why, I'm not quite sure, as the first food is anything *but* solid!). Weaning means the process of introducing food other than milk to your baby's diet and gradually winding down the milk-feeds. The whole process is expected to take about nine months.

New recommendations by the Department of Health in their report on 'Weaning and the Weaning Diet' indicate that babies should start to experience their first tastes of food at four months. This is different to previous government recommendations of three months, and in fact surveys show that many mothers have been introducing their babies to food even earlier.

From a survey conducted in 1986 by the Ministry of Agriculture, Fisheries and Food on a sample of 488 babies, it was discovered that by eight weeks of age 16 per cent of them had received solid food and by three months the proportion was 52 per cent. During the first four or five months of life, healthy babies double their birth weight, and reach the stage where they require more energy and nutrients than milk can supply. However, there are some very good reasons why we should wait for the right signs before introducing the baby to solids. Introducing them too

194

soon can create problems for the baby, not only in childhood, but also in later life. If the gut is not ready to deal with the new food, the baby may develop food intolerances and allergies, and in some cases even coeliac disease which is an allergy to foods containing gluten, like wheat, oats, barley and rye.

Here are a few other guidelines:

★ For a start the baby must be able to sit up, supported in a chair, in order to cope with swallowing a mouthful of food.
★ The digestive system and the kidneys have to be developed sufficiently to cope with different types of food, which does not usually occur until four months of age.
★ The baby himself must be ready to co-operate, showing signs of interest in food *you* are eating, for example. Some babies even attempt to take food that you are eating from your hand, or watch you eating and open their mouths just as you open yours!
★ If your baby is able to hold an object and get it to his mouth, that is a sign that he may be ready.
★ Your baby may start waking in the night after previously sleeping soundly, or might appear not to be fully satisfied after a good milk-feed.
★ Don't be swayed by the fact that baby-food manufacturers state that their food is suitable for three-month-old babies, let the research guide you instead.

Breast-fed babies are likely to enjoy new tastes and accept foods more readily than bottle-fed babies, probably because they have been used to a variety of different tastes in your breast-milk. Bottle-fed babies have only had one flavour on the menu!

The rate of development amongst babies does vary, so you will need to look for the signs. Being too late with the introduction of new foods to your baby can also be damaging, as his diet might have become deficient, failing to supply him with the amount of nutrients he needed. He could also develop co-ordination problems as a result of not being offered food to handle and swallow.

HOME-COOKED FOOD

In past generations women did not think twice about preparing their babies' meals themselves. These days the majority of us rely far too heavily on pre-prepared foods, and it seems that the same is true when it comes to weaning our babies. A survey of 1,000 new mums, conducted by the National Childbirth Trust in conjunction with the Health Visitors' Association, concluded that there is too much convenience food in our babies' diets. The survey found that:

★ 70 per cent of the mothers turned to baby-food manufacturers for advice on weaning
★ 74 per cent of the mums make up their babies' feed with 50 per cent convenience food
★ 70 per cent of breast-feeding counsellors believe that convenience foods account for a higher proportion of babies' diets than ever before
★ 68 per cent of health visitors believe that advertising, the media, and professional information have confused parents about the nutritional needs of their children
★ 43 per cent of mothers introduced solids under three months, with some admitting to introducing solids at only a few weeks

Babies prefer home-cooked food as the taste will be more varied than the shop-bought varieties. It is much cheaper in the long run to cook for your baby, and much more nourishing. Neither is it much bother when you are cooking for yourself and other members of the family as well. Once

you get into a routine it takes very little time to prepare
baby meals, and these days with freezers, once your baby is
eating reasonable amounts, you can store several meals after
one cooking session.

When you are cooking vegetables, just cook a few more,
and it's the same with fruit and, later, meat. Then, either
with a mincer or preferably a liquidiser, you can make up
your baby's meal. To begin with, it might only consist of
one type of food, but after a few weeks you will be mixing
foods like fruit and rice with a little breast- or formula milk,
or carrot and potato with a little meat. If you are freezing
food in ice-cube trays, don't forget to defrost some in time
for the baby's meal!

In the early stages, when he is only eating little tastes,
buying jars of food is a waste of money anyway. If you do
intend to buy baby food later on, then go for the organic
variety, which you can be sure is free of chemicals from the
soil. Many baby-food manufacturers produce an organic
range now, so shop around.

Feeding solids and giving breast-milk at the same meal
can slightly reduce the absorption of iron from the breast-
milk. So try and keep them separate as soon as is feasible.
However in the early stages this will be impossible.

How To Go About It

When you start offering your baby real food you will only
need to use very small amounts. Rather than buying pre-
prepared baby food, use some vegetables you are preparing
for dinner, but do not salt them before his portion has been
removed.

★ Give your baby the first half of his milk-feed, so that he
is feeling happy and sociable before you start.

197

★ Start with carrot, mashed or puréed, and mixed with a little breast-milk.

★ Make sure that all the utensils you use have been sterilised or washed until they are scrupulously clean.

★ Use a feeding spoon and a bib so that you don't soil his clothes.

★ Sit your baby on your lap, or in his chair facing you, and let him know that this is the big moment.

★ Put a small amount of carrot purée on the spoon and put it to his lips. If you open your mouth he is likely to copy you!

★ Just give him a little taste at first and watch for the funny faces he is likely to make.

★ If you are lucky enough to get a few spoons down, call it a day. Give him the rest of his milk-feed, and don't forget to tell him how clever he is.

★ If your baby didn't co-operate, don't feel upset, the chances are it's not your cooking, but simply that it is going to take him a little while to get the hang of it.

Feed your baby at meal-times so that he gets the idea that it's a family event. During the first few weeks I would suggest just offering him tastes of food at lunch-time. When you feel he is ready, he can have a taste at breakfast-time and dinner-time as well. It will take you a while to organise yourself, and to remember to feed him a mini-meal. Don't panic if it doesn't all go smoothly at first, he will soon cooperate and come to enjoy his food.

STAGE ONE FOODS

The first foods you offer a baby between the age of four to six months should be:

★ smooth in texture

★ mild in flavour
★ natural without any added sugar or salt
★ free of any additives, preservatives or artificial flavours.

You would be wise to stick closely to the first-stage foods for the first eight weeks, as these are the most commonly 'safe' foods that your baby is likely to be able to cope with. These include:

★ soft cooked puréed vegetables like carrot, potato, cabbage, sweet potato, parsnips or swede
★ soft cooked puréed fruit like apple, pear, or banana, melon, peach, nectarine, or ripe avocado
★ baby rice cereal or puréed rice
★ small amounts of puréed meat, or pulses can be tried at the end of this stage. Mix them with rice and vegetables.

You can add a small amount of cow's milk at this stage. Use formula cow's milk or follow-on milks to soften foods like banana. You can try a little plain full-fat yoghurt. If anyone in your family has an allergy to dairy products, leave them out altogether until your baby has reached at least six months.

USEFUL TIPS
★ Stronger tasting foods like cabbage, parsnips or Brussels sprouts may need to be mixed with some rice or potato to soften the flavour.
★ As your baby's iron stores are likely to be running low at this point, you should try to incorporate foods that contain good amounts of Vitamin C, like fruit and vegetables, which will aid the absorption of iron from the diet.
★ Make up tiny quantities of food in the initial stages. If you want to preserve it, try freezing it in an ice-cube tray,

then you can simply defrost a little at a time. If you are planning to freeze food, make sure you freeze it as soon as it has cooled down. Don't leave food for your baby uncovered.

★ Fruit and vegetables are a good source of fibre. Regular amounts will prevent your baby from becoming constipated.

★ Try one new food at a time. If it goes down well over a period of a few days it can stay on the menu. Then move on to try another food. Adding foods one at a time initially is a useful way of telling whether your baby likes the food and whether it agrees with him.

★ If your baby does develop a rash or tummy ache or a gut upset – sickness, constipation or diarrhoea – then remove the food that you think may be causing the problem and wait a few weeks before trying it again.

FINGER FOODS

Babies love to participate and, more than that, they love to get messy. When your baby is about five months old, he should be able to hold a piece of soft food in his hand and help himself to a little nibble. Make sure it is only soft food like a piece of cooked carrot or a slice of ripe peach, and sit with him. Never leave unattended a baby who is eating as he may choke.

WHAT YOUR BABY SHOULD BE DRINKING

During Stage One the only drink your baby needs is breast-milk or formula, which will provide the good nutrients he increasingly needs. If you start introducing other drinks you will fill him up on far less nutritious fluid, and will be doing him a disservice. Even if this stage coincides with a hot summer you should not be tempted to give him water, unless it's an occasional occurrence. When you are breast-feeding, the fore-milk is watery anyway, so there is certainly no need to give any additional drinks.

WHICH MILK AND WHEN

Ordinary whole cow's milk should not be used as a drink until your baby is one year of age. Semi-skimmed milk is not suitable for children under the age of two, provided their diet is nutritionally adequate. According to the latest Department of Health report on weaning, skimmed milk is not suitable for children under five. I would go a stage further and say that it is not suitable for children who are not overweight, full stop.

When you start to introduce whole cow's milk, you might like to choose the organic variety that is now available in most supermarkets.

Birth to 4 months	Breast-milk or formula feeds only. You can use soya based formula milk if allergic to cow's milk based ones.
From 4–6 months	Continue with breast-milk or formula feeds as before.
From 6–9 months	Continue with breast-milk or formula feeds. Add hard cheese like Cheddar and you can now use whole cow's milk to soften solids. You can add yoghurt and custard.
From 9–12 months	Continue with breast-milk or formula feeds, with hard cheeses, with whole cow's milk to soften solids, and with the yoghurt and custard.
From 1 year	Whole cow's milk can be used now as a drink. Lower-fat milk can be used in cooking only. Do not use skimmed milk, it is too low in fat and calories.
	Soya, goat's and sheep's milk can be used but some babies and infants are allergic to

these. Ask your doctor and health visitor
if need be.

SAMPLE BABY DIET, STAGE ONE

Continue breast-feeding or giving formula milk-feeds in the
usual quantities during Stage One.

WEEK 1
At lunch-time, after at least half of the milk-feed, offer your
baby some carrot purée from a feeding spoon. Blend a small
cooked carrot with a dessertspoon of breast-milk or formula
milk to form a smooth paste.

Repeat this each lunch-time for the first week, and don't
forget to give the other half of the milk-feed once the solids
are finished with.

WEEK 2
Again at lunch-time, after the first half of the milk-feed,
offer your baby a little baby rice. You can either purée some
cooked rice with a little breast- or formula milk, or buy a
packet of organic baby rice and mix up a little with the baby's
milk.

WEEK 3
This week you can increase the feeds to two per day – lunch-
time and dinner-time. You can add fresh apple purée made
from one eating apple and sweetened with concentrated
(agar-agar free) apple juice, if necessary.

Lunch   A few spoons of baby rice followed by a few spoons
of mashed banana or apple purée

Dinner A few spoons of carrot purée followed by apple purée or mashed banana

WEEK 4
If all is going well, and your baby is welcoming the tastes of solids, you can increase the portion sizes a little and put breakfast on the menu.

Breakfast Baby rice with apple or pear purée to follow

Lunch Sweet potato purée, with apple or pear purée or mashed banana to follow

Dinner Carrot and baby rice, with apple or pear purée or mashed banana to follow

WEEK 5
This week add in potato and well-cooked lean meat.

Breakfast Baby rice, followed by apple or pear purée

Lunch Carrot and meat purée, followed by apple or pear purée

Dinner Meat, potato and carrot purée followed by apple or pear purée or mashed banana

WEEK 6
This week, add in mashed avocado pear. Try also a peach purée, made from fresh peaches if they are in season; if not, use finely mashed melon or mango.

Breakfast Baby rice, followed by apple or pear purée or mashed banana

Lunch   Meat and sweet potato or potato and carrot purée, followed by mango, peach or melon purée

Dinner   Avocado pear mixed with a little baby rice at first to temper the strong flavour, followed by fruit purée (choose from those fruits already introduced)

WEEK 7
This week, provided you have no history of allergy to dairy products in your family, you can introduce your baby to a little natural yoghurt or *fromage frais*, and you could also add chicken.

Breakfast   Baby rice and fruit purée (from the list already introduced)

Lunch   Chicken, potato and carrot purée, followed by live natural yoghurt mixed with fruit purée or *fromage frais*

Dinner   Avocado pear purée with cooked carrot sticks as finger food, with fresh fruit purée or mashed banana to follow   .

WEEK 8
This week you can introduce some cooked and puréed dried apricots, and some sticks of Cheddar cheese as finger food.

Breakfast   Baby rice and fruit purée (from your tried and tested list)

Lunch   Puréed chicken, potato and carrot, followed by puréed cooked dried apricots

Dinner   Puréed lamb and sweet potato, followed by a favourite fruit purée

When you feel the meal routine has been established, and your baby has turned six months, you can move on to Stage Two.

CHAPTER 18

Weaning Stage Two:
From Six to Nine Months

By the time your baby has reached six months he will probably be able to hold food in his hands and will be learning to chew, regardless of whether any teeth have appeared yet. These skills should be encouraged as it is much harder to teach older babies to chew and to help themselves. By seven months he will have learned how to shut his mouth and turn his head – as well as the art of refusing food! If he consistently refuses a certain type of food, it may just mean he doesn't like it, or perhaps it doesn't agree with him.

Once these new skills are in place you can begin to add more foods into his diet, and the consistency can gradually become a little more lumpy. Most babies get a taste for lumpy food and then refuse the purée, so don't be surprised when this happens.

Survey of Mothers
WEANING HABITS

We analysed the questionnaires of 148 women taken from the original 652, whose babies were aged between 12 and 23 months simply because they would have had a chance to introduce a whole range of foods, whereas mothers with younger babies perhaps would not, and it was recent enough for them to be able to remember very accurately.

The average age for introduction of solids was 3.4 months. 44 women (30 per cent) introduced wheat before 16 weeks.

Formula/Cow's Milk   18 women (12%) had never used it. 58 (39%) introduced it at birth. A further 20 (13.5%) introduced it within the first month, and a further 17% had introduced it by the third month.

Soya Milk   20 women (13.5%) had introduced soya milk, 16 of them before trying cow's milk/formula.

Ordinary Cow's Milk/Yoghurt   9 women had not tried it. 5% introduced it before 4 months.

Meat   22 women (15%) had not tried it. 47% had tried it by 6 months, which rose to a total of 85% by one year. The earliest introduction of meat was 9 weeks.

Meat and Fish-based Meals   9% had not tried them. The earliest introduction was 8 weeks. 45% had introduced them by 4 months. A further 46% had introduced them by 9 months.

	When introduced
Solids	14.5 weeks
Baby formula milk	8.7 weeks
Baby formula soya milk	7.6 weeks
Fresh vegetables	17.5 weeks
Fresh fruit	18.0 weeks
Baby meal not containing meat/fish	15.6 weeks
Baby meal containing meat/fish	19.1 weeks
Ordinary cow's milk	37.7 weeks

Eggs	36.0 weeks
Meat	28.2 weeks
Rice	20.4 weeks
Wheat	19.9 weeks

The conclusions of this part of the survey are that many of the women, probably through ignorance, are giving solids too early, before their baby's system is mature enough to cope. Wheat was introduced at around four and a half months, when the recommended time would be after nine months. Ordinary cow's milk, which is not recommended as a drink for your baby until one year, was introduced at just under thirty-eight weeks.

EXTRA VITAMINS AND MINERALS NEEDED

By six months also, especially if your baby is being breast-fed, he will be running short of vitamins like A and D, and the important minerals iron and zinc. You will need to incorporate plenty of foods that have high levels of these nutrients in particular, as well as giving a vitamin and mineral supplement. There is a section on the nutritional content of foods which begins on page 241. Browse through those lists before working out the menu for your baby. If you are still breast-feeding it would be a good idea to work your own diet out from the lists as well, to ensure that you continue to get as many good nutrients as possible.

KEEP GOOD RECORDS

Your baby should now be having three meals a day, preferably at family meal-times. Even if you are not eating a main meal when you feed your baby, have a snack so that he can see that you are doing the same as he is. Babies love to mimic. By now he will be ready to try a whole selection of new foods, in addition to the Stage One foods he has already grown used to. Still utilise the principle of adding one new food to his diet at a time, and if all goes well add another flavour a few days later. It's useful to keep a chart of what has been tried: tick off the foods that were well accepted, and make a note about any foods that you felt dubious about.

If there is no history of allergy in your family the introduction of new foods should go pretty smoothly. However, if you or a close relative have an allergy, or sensitivity to a certain food or food group, I would suggest leaving this out of your baby's diet until he has reached nine months. By following this approach you will be giving your baby's gut time to mature further so that a possible allergic reaction is less likely to damage the lining of his gut.

STAGE TWO FOODS

In addition to the milk-feeds that your baby continues to have, and in addition to the Stage One foods, you can now add the following:

* ★ soft-cooked white fish, skinned and meticulously boned
* ★ hard cheese, like Cheddar, can be grated, or sliced as a finger food
* ★ wholemeal and white bread
* ★ small amounts of oat, millet, tapioca, corn and wheat-based cereals (one at a time)
* ★ soft raw fruits and vegetables like banana, melon and tomato can be used as finger foods
* ★ sliced hard-boiled egg, slices of bread without crusts,

peeled cucumber and fruits such as banana, apple and pear can be used as a finger food. Make sure that you only offer eggs with a hard yolk to prevent Salmonella infection
★ stick to breast-, formula milk or water as a drink – fruit juices are not necessary at this point. If you are offering water then present it in a baby cup, with a lid, so that he can get used to feeding himself from a cup.

USEFUL TIPS
★ Remember that, to improve iron absorption, you should give foods containing Vitamin C (fruit and vegetables) with every meal.
★ Use little or no added fat when you are cooking foods for your baby which already contain fat (meat, for instance). Make sure you trim the fat off meat before serving it.
★ Avoid adding fatty food or foods containing salt or sugar to your baby's diet.
★ Stick to your three meals per day, and discourage snacking until your baby is enjoying his meals.
★ Cereals derived from whole grains are a richer source of nutrients and fibre than refined cereals.
★ Many of the baby cereals are fortified with iron and Vitamin B – try to use these where possible.

SAMPLE BABY DIET, STAGE TWO

Your baby will need a similar amount of breast-milk or formula as he did in the first stage of weaning, perhaps slightly less, depending on his appetite.

By this stage you should be feeding your baby three solid meals per day, each consisting of two courses. Your baby will undoubtedly let you know if a new taste isn't acceptable, by pulling a face, turning his head or simply spitting the food out!

In Stage Two you can gradually introduce additional groups of more complex foods. The texture should still be on the fine side, only gradually consisting of little lumps, similar to cottage cheese.

WEEK 9 (from seven months)

Breakfast   Porridge with apple purée

Lunch   Avocado pear purée with carrot sticks, followed by mashed banana

Dinner   Beef, carrot, potato and cabbage puréed with the juices from the meat. Fruit, fruit purée or yoghurt for pudding.

WEEK 10 (from seven months)

Breakfast   Porridge with mashed pear

Lunch   Soft-cooked white fish flakes with mashed potato and carrot, followed by mashed peaches

Dinner   Finely minced chicken with sweet potato and cabbage purée, followed by *fromage frais* and small sticks of banana

WEEK 11 (from seven months)

Breakfast   Porridge with puréed dried apricots, plus small sticks of oatcake with a thin layer of Whole Earth sugar-free fruit spread

Lunch   Grated Cheddar cheese with tomato quarters, followed by rice pudding

Dinner   Finely minced beef, with courgettes, carrots and potato mashed with a little breast- or formula milk or meat juices, followed by mashed mango

WEEK 12 (from eight months)

Breakfast   Cornflakes softened with breast-milk or formula, plus banana soldiers

Lunch   Mashed lentils with well-cooked rice, followed by thinly cut peeled raw apple slices

Dinner   Soft-cooked white fish flakes with a mixture of mashed potato, mashed green beans and carrot, followed by baked apple and raisins

WEEK 13 (from eight months)

Breakfast   Hard-boiled egg and fingers of bread soldiers

Lunch   Baked potato mixed with mashed baked beans, followed by baked egg custard

Dinner   Minced chicken with mashed cauliflower and sweet potato, followed by cooked dried apricots, mashed and mixed with *fromage frais*

WEEK 14 (from nine months)

Breakfast   Weetabix softened with breast-milk or formula, plus banana soldiers

Lunch Chopped avocado pear with finely chopped tomato and cucumber, followed by rice pudding

Dinner Soya mince with finely chopped broccoli and potato, followed by baked or tinned pears in natural juice

WEEK 15 (from nine months)

Breakfast Rice Crispies softened with breast-milk or formula, plus chopped dried apricots

Lunch Home-made vegetable soup, followed by tapioca pudding

Dinner Braised beef with finely chopped carrot and parsnip, followed by finely cut apple slices with raisins

WEEK 16 (from nine months)

Breakfast Scrambled egg with wholemeal bread soldiers, plus stewed apple

Lunch Cauliflower cheese with baked potato, followed by fresh or tinned peaches in natural juice

Dinner Minestrone, followed by semolina with baked pear

WEEK 17 (from nine months)

Breakfast Puffed rice with breast-milk or formula, plus banana soldiers

Lunch Mashed lentils and mixed vegetables, followed by finely cut pear slices

Dinner Soft-cooked white fish flakes with mashed courgettes and tomatoes, followed by home-made fruit jelly

By now you should have a good idea of what your baby
likes and doesn't like. Continue to avoid those foods that
may have upset him or her. Mild reactions to foods are not
uncommon. You may find that a few months later the food
is tolerated. If there is a severe reaction, speak to your doctor
before trying it again.

CHAPTER 19

Weaning Stage Three:
From Nine to Twelve Months

At this stage your baby is likely to have cut a few teeth and will be well into communicating his likes and dislikes. He will be able to pick up his own food with his fingers or a feeding spoon, and will be generally making a lovely mess, especially if other members of the family laugh at his antics. This brings back wonderful memories of our elder son at meal-times at about nine or ten months. For some reason he thought that he should wash his hair with food, particularly sticky food. The more we showed our amusement, the more he performed. It became a standing joke in the family, and he went on to teach the younger two children how to develop the same technique!

As growth remains rapid at this stage in your baby's life, and he will be using up much more energy crawling, generally exploring and attempting to walk, it follows that his demand for nutrients will be even greater than before.

STAGE THREE FOODS

He should still be consuming more or less the same amount of milk, and in addition all the foods that you have introduced with success so far. If you have a list of foods that he rejected or that you were unsure about, this is the

215

time to reintroduce them, one at a time, to see whether he is ready to accept them.

In addition to all this he will now be ready to try a further list of foods.

★ You can continue to use whole cow's milk to mix solids, but don't give cow's milk as a drink until your baby is over a year old.
★ Starchy foods such as rice, potato and pasta can now be given in a drier form without added milk or juices.
★ Offer wholemeal bread and pasta products rather than white.
★ Introduce raw vegetables as finger foods, like sticks of carrot, cauliflower, celery, and cucumber. Segments of raw fruit like orange, satsuma or slices of mango or paw paw can be offered as well.
★ He can now drink unsweetened orange juice or apple juice at meal-times, but dilute it half and half with filtered or boiled water. Use a baby cup, with a lid, rather than a bottle.
★ You can use moderate amounts of butter or margarine and even small amounts of low-sugar or sugar-free jam on bread.

WHAT TO AVOID
★ Avoid adding any salt to food, and avoid large amounts of salty foods like Marmite or bacon. A young baby has a limited capacity to deal with a lot of salt. It can even raise its blood pressure!
★ Try to restrict your baby's intake of foods containing sugar.
★ Don't offer him any fizzy drinks, especially cola, or diet drinks.
★ Nuts are unsuitable for babies and children under five years of age, unless they are puréed, like peanut butter,

almond butter and so on. These make nutritious spreads, and are usually very popular with children. However, some children, especially those with eczema or asthma, are allergic to peanuts. If there has been one severe reaction, avoid them completely. Take note that peanut is included in many vegetarian packaged foods, e.g. vegeburgers.

★ Smoked and pickled foods are bad for young children so avoid them.

★ Young babies cannot usually tolerate spicy foods, so season your food after you have separated the baby's food.

SAMPLE BABY DIET, STAGE THREE

DAY 1

Breakfast Scrambled egg with melted Cheddar cheese ● Fruit yoghurt ● Small amount of diluted apple juice

Lunch Vegetable soup with rice ● Banana soldiers ● Small amount of diluted apple juice

Dinner Finely cut roast chicken, baked potato, cabbage and peas ● Baked apple with raisins ● Small amount of diluted apple juice

DAY 2

Breakfast Weetabix softened with whole cow's milk ● Chopped stewed dried apricots ● Small amount of diluted orange juice

Lunch   Celery, carrots and cucumber with lentil purée • Home-made fruit jelly • Small amount of diluted orange juice

Dinner   Lentil and vegetable bake • Apple crumble with custard

DAY 3

Breakfast   French toast • Banana soldiers • Small amount of diluted pineapple juice

Lunch   Chopped stir-fry vegetables and noodles • Peach slices

Dinner   Baked white fish with spinach and cheese sauce • Yoghurt with chopped fruit

DAY 4

Breakfast   Cornflakes mixed with whole cow's milk • *Fromage frais* • Small amount of diluted apple juice

Lunch   Cheese soldiers and raisins with tomato, cucumber and grated carrot • Satsuma

Dinner   Finely cut baked lamb with carrots, green beans and mashed potatoes • Baked banana

DAY 5

Breakfast   Cheerio oat cereal mixed with whole cow's milk • Stewed apple

Lunch   Baked spinach, egg and cheese • Kiwi fruit

Dinner Shepherd's pie (made with meat or soya mince) with cauliflower and peas ● Mango slices

DAY 6

Breakfast Jordan's muesli softened with whole cow's milk ● Satsuma

Lunch Pasta with cheese and tomato sauce ● Chopped grapes (without skins or pips)

Dinner Finely cut braised beef with broccoli, carrots and potato ● *Fromage frais* with pear slices

DAY 7

Breakfast Jordan's Oat Crunchy cereal softened with whole cow's milk ● Raw apple slices

Lunch Raw carrot, cauliflower and cucumber with hummus dip ● Baked egg custard

Dinner Tuna and pasta bake with peas and sweetcorn ● Melon slices

Your baby is now familiar with the majority of foods he's likely to be eating for the rest of his life. Sitting down to regular family meals will help him develop a healthy approach to eating and enjoying foods.

Chapter 20

Vegetarian Babies

Vegetarian babies can be just as healthy as meat eaters, but strict vegetarian parents need to be specially educated about how to meet their growing baby's nutritional needs. One of the problems with a vegetarian diet is that many of the foods are low in energy and bulky, resulting in the children not being able to consume large amounts. Additionally, many vegetarian foods such as bran and wholewheat contain high levels of phytic acid, which tends to impede the absorption of important minerals like iron, zinc and calcium. Phytates are found in the nutritious but hard-to-digest whole-grain cereal foods. Initially they should be added to the diet only in small amounts.

One way of helping to provide the baby with all that she needs is to choose foods that have a high Vitamin C content, as Vitamin C helps to enhance iron absorption. The presence of protein in the diet also increases iron absorption, probably because it combines with phytates and reduces their effect on iron absorption. Unfortunately, many vegetarian sources of protein contain far less protein from any single source when compared to animal protein, and unlike animal protein do not contain all the essential amino acids. These are needed for the development of muscle and other protein-rich tissues in the baby. Educated vegetarians can combine plant sources so that the full range of amino acids can more easily be obtained. Soya protein is a good source of amino acids and is therefore an important part of a vegetarian weaning diet. Good combinations are:

★ rice with beans or peas
★ wheat with beans or nuts and milk
★ nuts with sunflower seeds
★ soya with wheat and sesame
★ sweetcorn with beans or peas

During Stage One of the weaning process, between four and six months, small amounts of lentils, peas (ordinary frozen are fine), haricot beans or butter beans should be added to your baby's diet. They should be well cooked and softened with either breast-milk, formula or soya formula, and combined with rice. Include some fruit and vegetables in the same meal to improve the absorption of iron.

As the baby progresses to Stages Two and Three, fruit juice containing Vitamin C may be added to the diet, in addition to the fruit and vegetables, to aid iron absorption.

THE VEGAN DIET

Breast-fed babies who are born to vegan mothers in Great Britain, and weaned on a vegan diet, are reported to grow and develop normally, according to the Department of Health report on the 'Weaning and the Weaning Diet'. However, these children tend to be smaller and lighter than meat eaters as their diet contains less energy.

Once again a careful selection of vegetarian foods, including those that contain fats, should be selected in order to meet the growing baby's needs. As with vegetarians, it is also important to concentrate on fruit and vegetables with a high Vitamin C content, to help prevent the iron in the diet binding with the phytic acid present in many vegetarian and vegan foods.

A strict vegan diet cannot provide Vitamin B12 or adequate amounts of riboflavin, Vitamin B2. New-born babies born to well-nourished mothers will inherit stores of Vitamin B12 and riboflavin. Breast-fed babies will also be protected for a period of time, but supplements of both vitamins will be needed. It is advisable for vegan babies to be breast-fed for as long as possible, and then to be weaned on to soya milk.

You will find the address of both the Vegetarian and Vegan Society in the appendix on page 281. It will undoubtedly have further advice to offer.

CHAPTER 21

Food Allergy and Intolerance

There is no doubt that certain foods and drinks produce adverse and sometimes very unpleasant symptoms in some people. When these symptoms recur every time the person eats or drinks a particular food, they are usually termed food allergies. Strictly speaking, the term food allergy should be reserved for situations where the body's immune system is affected. Only a small percentage of people have true allergies: the majority, who genuinely react to foods, suffer with *food intolerances*, which are sometimes transient depending on the nutritional state that the individual is in at the time.

Allergic reactions to food seem to be increasingly common. Eczema, asthma, rhinitis, catarrh, migraine and bowel problems can all be triggered by food allergy or intolerance. Food intolerances may be due to a number of physiological factors, including the presence of toxins which can irritate the lining of the gut, the lack of an ability to produce a particular enzyme needed for the digestion of that food, a drug-like effect from caffeine for example, or simply discomfort due to unabsorbed food residues in the gut.

Surveys show that as many as two in ten people in Britain believe that they react to certain foods in their diet, although estimates of the actual number of people who are intolerant varies considerably. A government study, for example, suggests that less than two out of every hundred people

223

suffer with a reaction that can actually be measured scientifically.

Babies are more likely to react to foods because their immature gut is not ready to deal with a particular type of food, like wheat or cow's milk. It is thought that about one in ten young children is affected by food in some way, but as many as 80 per cent of these grow out of the intolerance by the time they are five years old.

THE SYMPTOMS LINKED WITH ALLERGY

A wide variety of complaints can be due to food allergy. In general many allergic complaints have nearly trebled in frequency since the Second World War. Care is needed in making the diagnosis as all the conditions that follow can be caused by other factors.

★ Gut symptoms, which may include abdominal pain, wind, toddler-diarrhoea, constipation and even infantile colitis.
★ Skin outbreaks like eczema or urticaria (nettle rash or hives).
★ Nose and chest symptoms from catarrh and a runny nose at one end of the spectrum to asthma at the other.
★ Behavioural changes – hyperactivity in children, mood swings and aggression in adults, for example.
★ Migraine headaches.
★ Arthritis.
★ And, in rare cases, systemic reactions like anaphylactic shock, which leads to swelling in the throat, a sudden drop in blood pressure, and can result in death if not treated quickly with adrenaline.

224

WHICH FOODS CAN CAUSE REACTIONS?

It is usually the common foods which cause the most problems.

★ milk and cheese
★ wheat and other grains
★ fish and shellfish
★ nuts and peanuts
★ colouring agents
★ soya products
★ eggs
★ pork or bacon
★ chocolate
★ citrus fruits like oranges, satsumas and grapefruit
★ tea and coffee
★ food preservatives
★ strawberries

The very small minority of people who have a severe reaction, which requires the use of adrenaline on an emergency basis, usually react to nuts or shellfish. If there is any history of such severe allergy in your family you should undoubtedly inform your doctor and be supervised by your local paediatric dietician.

Case History

Barbara had been seen a year before because of her premenstrual symptoms. These had improved when she changed her diet and had taken supplements of multi-vitamins and magnesium.

She had subsequently relaxed the diet a little without immediate ill-effect, and now was pregnant. The first four months were a trial. In the first month she had 'flu' and had not felt well since. Vomiting began with the 'flu', and continued, resulting in a weight loss of half a stone. She was severely troubled by abdominal discomfort after eating, and because of her problems had spent several weeks in hospital. At eighteen weeks she was still underweight and had early signs that suggested a lack of Vitamin B – redness and greasiness at the sides of the nose and some redness at the tip of the tongue. Blood tests showed a low level of Vitamin B6 and other nutrients. Supplements of Vitamin B, dietary advice to eat little and often and to concentrate on nutritious easy-to-digest food, helped somewhat but she never felt really well and her appetite was always poor.

A further problem was that by thirty weeks she was anaemic and was not responding to supplements of iron. Poor absorption of her iron supplement was a possibility. A test for allergy to wheat and other grains was positive and she began a gluten-free diet. This meant avoiding all wheat, oats, barley and rye as well as any food containing them. There was a substantial improvement in her health. Her blood count improved, her appetite increased, and she lost her residual abdominal discomfort.

When she ate any bread, especially wholemeal, she noticed a return of her abdominal symptoms.

Her son was born at forty weeks and weighed 3 kg (7 lb).

Her sensitivity to wheat and other grains was probably evolving before and during her pregnancy. The diet that had helped her premenstrual problems had caused her to reduce her consumption of these grains and their reintroduction may equally have aggravated her morning sickness.

Reactions to Cow's Milk

There are two distinctly different ways that cow's milk can upset us. One is an intolerance to lactose, the milk sugar, and the other is a reaction to the protein in milk. They can produce similar symptoms and there are different ways of treating them.

REACTION TO LACTOSE

Lactose is a sugar that is present in both human milk and the milk of other animals. In order to be digested, it requires adequate amounts of an enzyme called lactase, which breaks the lactose down into simpler sugars which the body can then absorb. When an individual has insufficient levels of lactase to break down the lactose, it passes into the large intestine and causes symptoms like colic pain, wind and diarrhoea. This deficiency is more common among people from other parts of the world like South-East Asia, India, the Middle East and parts of Africa. It can also occur temporarily following an episode of infective gastroenteritis when giving a lot of milk can prolong the diarrhoea. Probably only 5 per cent of white British people have a lactase deficiency.

Many of those with lactase deficiency can tolerate small amounts of cow's milk without feeling any discomfort. Studies have shown that fermented milk products such as yoghurt and hard cheese are usually well tolerated in those with low lactase levels, even when milk is not. Research carried out at the University of Minnesota concluded that the lactose in live yoghurt was better absorbed than lactose in milk, and suggested that lactase produced by the bacteria in yoghurt may aid the digestion of lactose in the intestine. Another benefit of eating lactose-containing foods as part of a meal means that the emptying of your stomach is slowed down, which allows your gut more time to deal with the food.

A lactase preparation derived from yeast has been developed which, when combined with milk before it is consumed, splits the majority of the lactose into simple sugars, making it more acceptable to the gut.

REACTION TO MILK PROTEIN

Reacting to the protein in milk is probably less common than lactase deficiency, and more commonly occurs in babies who have a family history of allergy. The symptoms include sickness, diarrhoea, tummy pain and wind (similar to the symptoms mentioned for lactose intolerance), but skin symptoms like eczema, urticaria, and possibly cradle cap, as well as catarrh, are also possibly associated with milk protein allergy.

Fortunately, many children who experience milk protein allergy initially do grow out of it by the time they reach the age of five. In the meantime there are a number of measures to try.

★ If you are still breast-feeding, you can express some extra milk to mix with solids and delay the inclusion of cow's milk products into your baby's diet.

★ Try using soya milk formula instead, and later ordinary soya milk to see whether your baby can tolerate that any better. This is a controversial area at the moment, and although studies have shown that soya milk is not tolerated any better than cow's milk, that is not my experience. In fact two of our own children had a temporary intolerance to cow's milk and tolerated soya milk very well.

★ For infants who cannot tolerate cow's milk products, a formula milk based on hydrolysed milk protein is available on prescription, but some children cannot tolerate this either.

★ As time goes by you can try introducing small amounts of cow's milk or, better still, cow's milk products like live natural yoghurt and hard cheese.

★ Make sure you are giving your baby sufficient calcium and iron – check the food lists on page 241.

★ Liaise with your doctor or your health visitor so that they are aware of the difficulties you are having with your baby's diet.

DO FOOD INTOLERANCES RUN IN FAMILIES?

Genetic factors are known to contribute to allergies, and the risk of your baby developing an allergic disorder more than doubles if there is a family history of allergy. True allergies like asthma and eczema do seem to run in families. If both parents suffer from these allergic conditions, this greatly raises the chance of their offspring being so affected. A study from specialists on the Isle of Wight showed that attention to the mother's diet during pregnancy and in the first year of life can halve the chance of allergic disease developing in the baby by the time he reaches his first birthday. In this study of families where one or both parents suffered from eczema and other allergies, the mothers excluded milk, eggs, wheat and other foods from their diet during pregnancy, and whilst breast-feeding, and delayed their introduction into the babies' diets. By the time the babies were one year old, only half the expected number were suffering from eczema. Careful dietetic advice is needed when following these restricted diets.

If you have a known allergy, it is important to get it under control before you attempt to conceive. Many researchers now believe that you should avoid the foods to which you are intolerant right through from the preconceptual phase to the point when you stop breast-feeding. However, some women who have existing allergies before pregnancy are aware that these improve during pregnancy, possibly due to the positive changes in the immune system. This honeymoon period may end all too suddenly after birth with the return of allergic symptoms like asthma or eczema, but you can prolong it for a while if you are breast-feeding.

In order to protect your child it is advisable to go on breast-feeding for at least six months. When you begin weaning, omit the suspect foods from your baby's diet until she has reached at least six months, and preferably nine months to a year. By giving your baby's gut more chance to mature, she will be better able to deal with the suspect foods when you do introduce them.

Children who are on restricted diets are much more likely to suffer with deficiencies and fail to thrive so well unless the excluded food, especially milk with its high calcium content, is adequately compensated for.

HAS YOUR BABY DEVELOPED A FOOD INTOLERANCE?

When your baby goes from being contented to miserable and appears to be uncomfortable, she is either teething, sickening for something, or something in your milk or her food has upset her. If you are breast-feeding her exclusively, you will need to put on your nutritional detective hat, and list everything that has passed your lips for a few days to see if you can work out what is causing the problem. If she is in the process of being weaned, then you will need to try to think back to see whether you have recently introduced anything new into her diet. Once you have an idea what might be causing the problem, leave it out of your diet, and hers if necessary, for a few days and see whether she returns to her former happy self.

A lack of important nutrients like zinc and iron, and a

number of environmental factors, could undermine her
immune system and make her more susceptible to allergy.

★ If you are taking the pill and breast-feeding you should
look at using another contraceptive measure until you
finish breast-feeding. Residues of the pill hormones in
breast-milk can reduce her immunity.
★ Keep her away from smoky rooms, and make a point of
not letting anyone smoke anywhere near her at home.
★ If you live near a busy road, make sure you have fine net
curtains on the windows to reduce the fumes that come
into the house, or consider moving.
★ Wash all fruit and vegetables thoroughly before offering
them to her, and provide her with only organic fruits and
vegetables, either from the supermarket, a local market
or the home-grown variety. They will be free of chemicals.

Are Allergy Tests Worthwhile?

A variety of tests do exist to determine whether an individual
has an allergy. There are immunological tests, skin-prick tests
and some other tests which are of dubious scientific value.
The best way to confirm that your baby has an allergy or
intolerance is by doing a challenge test yourself. Remove
the food you suspect is causing a problem from her diet,
wait for the symptoms to calm down, and then reintroduce
the food and watch. If the symptoms recur you have
confirmed the problem for yourself.

There is no need to assume that 'once allergic, always
allergic', unless there is a strong family history of a particular
allergy. It is wise to make other dietary contingency plans
to ensure your baby continues to be well nourished, and
then attempt to reintroduce small amounts of the offending
food a few months later. Some studies have suggested that

in order to establish a normal immune response it is highly preferable to introduce the food you have been excluding back into the diet gradually.

If you are at all concerned don't hesitate to get some professional help.

CHAPTER 22

Look After *Yourself*

Not looking after yourself after your baby is born can have severe repercussions on your health. When you have been on the night-shift for several months, feeding on demand, and perhaps not having sufficient time to rest during the day when your baby does, you may begin to experience some undesirable health problems.

Some women just feel 'wiped out' physically, wishing they could sleep for a week. Others get irritable and moody, and their libido goes out the window, particularly once their periods have begun again. On the whole breast tenderness tends to improve after pregnancy.

The women in our survey, as you might expect, experienced a cross section of problems. We looked at a group of 250 women whose babies were age six to fourteen months.

Survey of 250 Mothers
AFTER PREGNANCY

	Same	Better	Worse	Never suffered	No reply
Fatigue	64	6	135	37	8
Low libido	65	12	91	71	11

Survey of 250 Mothers
PMS AND PERIOD SYMPTOMS AFTER LAST PREGNANCY

	No reply	Never	Same	Better	Worse
Moodiness	11	65	89	25	60
Tender breasts	11	125	67	32	15
Period pain	15	68	67	53	47
Heavy periods	17	71	70	27	65

CHANGES AFTER CHILDBIRTH

In my experience it's not just a question of getting your physical shape back after you've had a baby, there is the question of the little grey matter. I can remember going to the local supermarket about six weeks after I'd had our first baby, and I suddenly couldn't remember what I'd gone there for. I didn't see the funny side at the time, but got tearful and left in a hurry. Then there was that time that I was in the middle of a conversation and I honestly couldn't remember what I was talking about! Alan got quite used to me stopping mid sentence and waiting for him to remind me what we were talking about.

This may sound highly amusing, but for a normally organised and reasonably intelligent 28-year-old it was very upsetting. At first I was too afraid to talk to anyone about it as I thought it might be pre-senile dementia! When I did pluck up the courage to bring the subject up at a 'mothers' ' meeting I was somewhat relieved to discover I was not alone. From then on, after my babies were born, I referred to it as my 'out-to-lunch syndrome'! Fortunately the memory does return to some extent, but I would take quite some convincing that it ever returns completely.

Interestingly, some researchers at Bristol Maternity Hospital have at last begun to take seriously this loss of memory during and after pregnancy. A study conducted on sixty-seven women was divided into three groups, some of whom were newly pregnant, some pregnant who had previously had children, and others who were not pregnant. The pregnant women had much more difficulty remembering words they had just heard, compared to the non-pregnant women who remembered nearly double the number of words. The study also discovered that the women who had had several children had even lower scores than those who were pregnant for the first time! It seems that these lapses in memory are likely to be related to the dramatic increase in circulating progesterone during pregnancy.

If you do fall victim to the out-to-lunch syndrome, I suggest that you write yourself little notes.

★ Carry a little pad with you and write down everything that you need to remember as it occurs to you.
★ Keep a running check-list of things you have to do – just like a shopping list.
★ Let people around you know that you are feeling absent-minded.
★ Keep a note of important facts, like names, addresses and telephone numbers in your bag.
★ Spend a little time each day relaxing.
★ And most of all, don't panic, you will get your brain back!

So far as breasts are concerned, the good news is that breast-feeding a baby gives that child a better start in life, and also reduces your chances of getting breast cancer later in life. However, the bad news is that breasts do tend to change their shape and become saggy when you have fed a few children for any length of time. Exercising helps to keep the supporting muscles toned up, but in reality there is little you can do to get your nipples pointing up to the sky again. That seems to be the trade-off for producing lovely healthy babies.

Apart from the loss of memory and the fallen breasts, my hair fell out in handfuls, a hormonal reaction which prompted yet another panic. You would imagine that being a medical family, we would have anticipated these events. Not so at all, we didn't even know about them. That's how well the secret is kept! Why we are not forewarned about all these changes remains a mystery until this day. I am sure I would have coped and maintained a much greater sense of humour had I known what to expect, which is why I'm sharing this with you now.

Mother Nature, as we have discovered, is a wise old lady, so it stands to reason that each of the phenomena that present themselves along the way occur for a reason. For example, we put on excess weight during a normal pregnancy with the view of converting it into breast-milk once the baby is born. My theory about the memory loss is that we are designed to concentrate on the needs of our new baby and not to continue working, or over-extending ourselves in intellectual terms in those initial few months. Just as we get the nesting urge prior to delivery, so it follows that we should inhabit the nest for some time. I didn't even want to watch the news or read a newspaper for the few months after our babies were born. Any tragedy, no matter how small or distant, would make me feel exceedingly emotional. I just wanted uninterrupted family time, and to remain in 'cloud cuckoo land'. Don't assume I was suffering with post-natal depression, not at all; I was feeling fulfilled and happy to remain oblivious.

We estimate that it takes some five months for the hormones to settle down after pregnancy, and each time in my case it was a full year before I really felt that I'd got both my body and mind back again. The hormones go through massive and rapid changes adjusting to a pregnancy and then afterwards, allowing you to get back to normal. There are lots of things that you can do which will ease the passage. For a start, eating an exceptionally healthy diet will encourage both normal hormone function and brain chemical metabolism. Exercise will not only help you back to physical shape, but also has a very profound effect on brain chemicals as well as hormones. Taking a multi-vitamin and multi-mineral each day, especially if you are breast-feeding, will also aid your recovery.

When a month has passed since the baby was born you need to work out what I heard someone refer to as a 'ME' programme. This involves working out a self-enhancement routine that you can feasibly stick to. Try some of the following.

★ Work out a menu for yourself for a whole week. Then write a shopping list and ask your partner to do the honours. If you have him well trained he may even cook for you!

★ Bearing in mind your baby's routine, work out roughly when you could do a session of exercise, either a video at home, or have someone watch the baby whilst you go for a swim.

★ Once or twice per week, persuade a close family member or friend to watch your baby while you have an hour or two to yourself. Go out for a walk, do some shopping, or put your feet up with the knowledge that you are not going to be disturbed.

★ Get your hair cut and styled so that you feel better about looking in the mirror.

★ If you can afford it, buy a few new clothes, so that you feel a little more attractive.

237

★ Make sure you have time alone with your partner when you can talk about things other than nappies and other absorbing matters relating to your baby's routine.

When time has passed and you are back in good physical and mental shape you will find that the memory of labour and those sleepless nights begins to fade. It is even likely that your growing baby will be a source of so much joy that you will go on to have more children, realising that the down side to pregnancy and breast-feeding is only a temporary state of affairs. In the long term the one thing that most parents agree upon is that these small, all-consuming little bundles do provide us with constant pleasure, and the love that results from the relationship is beyond description.

Savour your child-bearing days, but do not forget to look after yourself. At the end of the day, your family will probably regard you as some kind of superwoman, who can and should fulfil their every need. If you intend to meet the challenge, you owe it to yourself as well as to them to remain in good shape so that you can give them the support they need, whilst still enjoying your rôle as a mother and lover.

APPENDICES

APPENDIX I

Nutritional Content of Foods

Unless stated otherwise, foods listed are raw

VITAMIN A – RETINOL
  Micrograms per 100 g (3.5 oz)

Skimmed milk	1
Semi-skimmed milk	21
Grilled herring	49
Whole milk	52
Porridge made with milk	56
Cheddar cheese	325
Margarine	800
Butter	815
Lamb's liver	15,000

VITAMIN B1 – THIAMIN
  Milligrams per 100 g (3.5 oz)

Peaches	0.02
Cottage cheese	0.02
Cox's apple	0.03
Full-fat milk	0.04
Skimmed milk	0.04
Semi-skimmed milk	0.04
Cheddar cheese	0.04
Bananas	0.04
White grapes	0.04
French beans	0.04
Low-fat yoghurt	0.05

Cantaloupe melon	0.05
Tomato	0.06
Green peppers, raw	0.07
Boiled egg	0.08
Roast chicken	0.08
Grilled cod	0.08
Haddock, steamed	0.08
Roast turkey	0.09
Mackerel, cooked	0.09
Savoy cabbage, boiled	0.10
Oranges	0.10
Brussels sprouts	0.10
Lentils, boiled	0.11
Potatoes, new, boiled	0.11
Soya beans, boiled	0.12
Red peppers, raw	0.12
Lentils, boiled	0.14
Steamed salmon	0.20
Corn	0.20
White spaghetti, boiled	0.21
Almonds	0.24
White self-raising flour	0.30
Plaice, steamed	0.30
Bacon, cooked	0.35
Walnuts	0.40
Wholemeal flour	0.47
Lamb's kidney	0.49
Brazil nuts	1.00
Cornflakes	1.00
Rice Krispies	1.00
Wheatgerm	2.01

VITAMIN B2-RIBOFLAVIN
Milligrams per 100 g (3.5 oz)

Cabbage, boiled	0.01
Potatoes, boiled	0.01
Brown rice, boiled	0.02
Pear	0.03
Wholemeal spaghetti, boiled	0.03
White self-raising flour	0.03
Orange	0.04
Spinach, boiled in salted water	0.05
Baked beans	0.06
Banana	0.06
White bread	0.06
Green peppers, raw	0.08
Lentils, boiled	0.08
Hovis	0.09
Soya beans, boiled	0.09
Wholemeal bread	0.09
Wholemeal flour	0.09
Peanuts	0.10
Baked salmon	0.11
Red peppers, raw	0.15
Full-fat milk	0.17
Avocado	0.18
Grilled herring	0.18
Semi-skimmed milk	0.18
Roast chicken	0.19
Roast turkey	0.21
Cottage cheese	0.26
Soya flour	0.31
Boiled prawns	0.34
Boiled egg	0.35
Topside of beef, cooked	0.35
Leg of lamb, cooked	0.38
Cheddar cheese	0.40
Muesli	0.70
Almonds	0.75
Cornflakes	1.50
Rice Krispies	1.50

VITAMIN B3 – NIACIN
Milligrams per 100 g (3.5 oz)

Boiled egg	0.07
Cheddar cheese	0.07
Full-fat milk	0.08
Skimmed milk	0.09
Semi-skimmed milk	0.09
Cottage cheese	0.13
Cox's apple	0.20
Cabbage, boiled	0.30
Orange	0.40
Baked beans	0.50
Potatoes, boiled	0.50
Soya beans, boiled	0.50
Lentils, boiled	0.60
Banana	0.70
Tomato	1.00
Avocado	1.10
Green peppers, raw	1.10
Brown rice	1.30
Wholemeal spaghetti, boiled	1.30
White self-raising flour	1.50
Grilled cod	1.70
White bread	1.70
Soya flour	2.00
Red peppers, raw	2.20
Almonds	3.10
Grilled herring	4.00
Wholemeal bread	4.10
Hovis	4.20
Wholemeal flour	5.70
Muesli	6.50
Topside of beef, cooked	6.50
Leg of lamb, cooked	6.60
Baked salmon	7.00
Roast chicken	8.20
Roast turkey	8.50
Boiled prawns	9.50
Peanuts	13.80
Cornflakes	16.00
Rice Krispies	16.00

VITAMIN B6 – PYRIDOXINE
Milligrams per 100 g (3.5 oz)

Carrots	0.05
Full-fat milk	0.06
Skimmed milk	0.06
Semi-skimmed milk	0.06
Satsuma	0.07
White bread	0.07
White rice	0.07
Cabbage, boiled	0.08
Cottage cheese	0.08
Cox's apple	0.08
Wholemeal pasta	0.08
Frozen peas	0.09
Spinach, boiled	0.09
Cheddar cheese	0.10
Orange	0.10
Broccoli	0.11
Hovis	0.11
Baked beans	0.12
Boiled egg	0.12
Red kidney beans, cooked	0.12
Wholemeal bread	0.12
Tomatoes	0.14
Almonds	0.15
Cauliflower	0.15
Brussels sprouts	0.19
Sweetcorn, boiled	0.21
Leg of lamb, cooked	0.22
Grapefruit juice	0.23
Roast chicken	0.26
Lentils, boiled	0.28
Banana	0.29
Brazil nuts	0.31
Potatoes, boiled	0.32
Roast turkey	0.33
Grilled herring	0.33
Topside of beef, cooked	0.33
Avocado	0.36
Grilled cod	0.38
Baked salmon	0.57

Soya flour	0.57
Hazelnuts	0.59
Peanuts	0.59
Walnuts	0.67
Muesli	1.60
Cornflakes	1.80
Rice Krispies	1.80
Special K	2.20

VITAMIN B12
Micrograms per 100 g (3.5 oz)

Tempeh	0.10
Miso	0.20
Quorn	0.30
Full-fat milk	0.40
Skimmed milk	0.40
Semi-skimmed milk	0.40
Marmite	0.50
Cottage cheese	0.70
Choux buns	1.00
Eggs, boiled	1.00
Eggs, poached	1.00
Halibut, steamed	1.00
Lobster, boiled	1.00
Sponge cake	1.00
Turkey, white meat	1.00
Waffles	1.00
Cheddar cheese	1.20
Eggs, scrambled	1.20
Squid	1.30
Eggs, fried	1.60
Shrimps, boiled	1.80
Parmesan cheese	1.90
Beef, lean	2.00
Cod, baked	2.00
Cornflakes	2.00
Pork, cooked	2.00
Raw beef mince	2.00
Rice Krispies	2.00
Steak, lean, grilled	2.00
Edam cheese	2.10
Eggs, whole, battery	2.40
Milk, dried, whole	2.40
Milk, dried, skimmed	2.60
Eggs, whole, free-range	2.70
Kambu seaweed	2.80
Squid, frozen	2.90
Taramasalata	2.90
Duck, cooked	3.00

Turkey, dark meat	3.00
Grapenuts	5.00
Tuna in oil	5.00
Herring, cooked	6.00
Herring roe, fried	6.00
Steamed salmon	6.00
Bovril	8.30
Mackerel, fried	10.00
Rabbit, stewed	10.00
Cod's roe, fried	11.00
Pilchards canned in tomato juice	12.00
Oysters, raw	15.00
Nori seaweed	27.50
Sardines in oil	28.00
Lamb's kidney, fried	79.00

FOLATE/FOLIC ACID
Micrograms per 100 g (3.5 oz)

Cox's apple	4.00
Leg of lamb, cooked	4.00
Full-fat milk	6.00
Skimmed milk	6.00
Semi-skimmed milk	6.00
Porridge with semi-skimmed milk	7.00
Turnip, baked	8.00
Sweet potato, boiled	8.00
Cucumber	9.00
Grilled herring	10.00
Roast chicken	10.00
Avocado	11.00
Grilled cod	12.00
Banana	14.00
Roast turkey	15.00
Carrots	17.00
Sweet potato	17.00
Tomatoes	17.00
Topside of beef, cooked	17.00
Swede, boiled	18.00
Strawberries	20.00
Brazil nuts	21.00
Red peppers, raw	21.00
Green peppers, raw	23.00
Rye bread	24.00
Dates, fresh	25.00
New potatoes, boiled	25.00
Grapefruit	26.00
Oatcakes	26.00
Cottage cheese	27.00
Baked salmon	29.00
Cabbage, boiled	29.00
Onions, boiled	29.00
White bread	29.00
Orange	31.00
Baked beans	33.00
Cheddar cheese	33.00
Clementines	33.00

Raspberries	33.00
Satsuma	33.00
Blackberries	34.00
Rye crispbread	35.00
Potato, baked in skin	36.00
Radish	38.00
Boiled egg	39.00
Hovis	39.00
Wholemeal bread	39.00
Red kidney beans, boiled	42.00
Potato, baked	44.00
Frozen peas	47.00
Almonds	48.00
Parsnips, boiled	48.00
Cauliflower	51.00
Green beans, boiled	57.00
Broccoli	64.00
Walnuts	66.00
Artichoke	68.00
Hazelnuts	72.00
Spinach, boiled	90.00
Brussels sprouts	110.00
Peanuts	110.00
Muesli	140.00
Sweetcorn, boiled	150.00
Asparagus	155.00
Chickpeas	180.00
Lamb's liver, fried	240.00
Cornflakes	250.00
Rice Krispies	250.00
Calf's liver, fried	320.00

VITAMIN C
Milligrams per 100 g (3.5 oz)

Full-fat milk	1.00
Skimmed milk	1.00
Semi-skimmed milk	1.00
Red kidney beans	1.00
Carrots	2.00
Cucumber	2.00
Muesli with dried fruit	2.00
Apricots, raw	6.00
Avocado	6.00
Pear	6.00
Potato, boiled	6.00
Spinach, boiled	8.00
Cox's apple	9.00
Turnip	10.00
Banana	11.00
Frozen peas	12.00
Lamb's liver, fried	12.00
Pineapple	12.00
Dried skimmed milk	13.00
Gooseberries	14.00
Raw dates	14.00
Melon	17.00
Tomatoes	17.00
Cabbage, boiled	20.00
Canteloupe melon	26.00
Cauliflower	27.00
Satsuma	27.00
Peach	31.00
Raspberries	32.00
Bran flakes	35.00
Grapefruit	36.00
Mangoes	37.00
Nectarine	37.00
Kumquats	39.00
Broccoli	44.00
Lychees	45.00
Unsweetened apple juice	49.00
Orange	54.00

Kiwi fruit	59.00
Brussels sprouts	60.00
Strawberries	77.00
Blackcurrants	115.00

VITAMIN D
Micrograms per 100g (3.5 oz)

Skimmed milk	0.01
Whole milk	0.03
Fromage frais	0.05
Cheddar cheese	0.26
Cornflakes	2.80
Rice Krispies	2.80
Kellogg's Start	4.20
Margarine	8.00

VITAMIN E
Milligrams per 100 g (3.5 oz)

Semi-skimmed milk	0.03
Boiled potatoes	0.06
Cucumber	0.07
Cottage cheese	0.08
Full-fat milk	0.09
Cabbage, boiled	0.10
Leg of lamb, cooked	0.10
Cauliflower	0.11
Roast chicken	0.11
Frozen peas	0.18
Red kidney beans, cooked	0.20
Wholemeal bread	0.20
Orange	0.24
Topside of beef, cooked	0.26
Banana	0.27
Brown rice, boiled	0.30
Grilled herring	0.30
Lamb's liver, fried	0.32
Baked beans	0.36
Cornflakes	0.40
Pear	0.50
Cheddar cheese	0.53
Carrots	0.56
Lettuce	0.57
Cox's apple	0.59
Grilled cod	0.59
Rice Krispies	0.60
Plums	0.61
Unsweetened orange juice	0.68
Leeks	0.78
Sweetcorn, boiled	0.88
Brussels sprouts	0.90
Broccoli	1.10
Boiled egg	1.11
Tomato	1.22
Watercress	1.46
Parsley	1.70
Spinach, boiled	1.71

Olives	1.99
Butter	2.00
Onions, dried raw	2.69
Mushrooms, fried in corn oil	2.84
Avocado	3.20
Muesli	3.20
Walnuts	3.85
Peanut butter	4.99
Olive oil	5.10
Sweet potato, baked	5.96
Brazil nuts	7.18
Peanuts	10.09
Pine nuts	13.65
Rapeseed oil	18.40
Almonds	23.96
Hazelnuts	24.98
Sunflower oil	48.70

CALCIUM
Milligrams per 100 g (3.5 oz)

Cox's apple	4.00
Brown rice, boiled	4.00
Potatoes, boiled	5.00
Banana	6.00
Topside of beef, cooked	6.00
White pasta, boiled	7.00
Tomato	7.00
White spaghetti, boiled	7.00
Leg of lamb, cooked	8.00
Red peppers, raw	8.00
Roast chicken	9.00
Roast turkey	9.00
Avocado	11.00
Pear	11.00
Butter	15.00
Cornflakes	15.00
White rice, boiled	18.00
Grilled cod	22.00
Lentils, boiled	22.00
Baked salmon	29.00
Green peppers, raw	30.00
Young carrots	30.00
Grilled herring	33.00
Wholemeal flour	38.00
Turnips, baked	45.00
Orange	47.00
Baked beans	48.00
Wholemeal bread	54.00
Boiled egg	57.00
Peanuts	60.00
Cottage cheese	73.00
Soya beans, boiled	83.00
White bread	100.00
Full-fat milk	115.00
Hovis	120.00
Muesli	120.00
Skimmed milk	120.00
Semi-skimmed milk	120.00

Prawns, boiled	150.00
Spinach, boiled	150.00
Brazil nuts	170.00
Yoghurt, low-fat, plain	190.00
Soya flour	210.00
Almonds	240.00
White self-raising flour	450.00
Sardines	550.00
Sprats, fried	710.00
Cheddar cheese	720.00
Whitebait, fried	860.00

IRON

Milligrams per 100 g (3.5 oz)

Semi-skimmed milk	0.05
Skimmed milk	0.06
Full-fat milk	0.06
Cottage cheese	0.10
Orange	0.10
Cox's apple	0.20
Pear	0.20
White rice	0.20
Banana	0.30
Cabbage, boiled	0.30
Cheddar cheese	0.30
Avocado	0.40
Grilled cod	0.40
Potatoes, boiled	0.40
Young carrots, boiled	0.40
Brown rice, boiled	0.50
Tomato	0.50
White pasta, boiled	0.50
Baked salmon	0.80
Roast chicken	0.80
Roast turkey	0.90
Grilled herring	1.00
Red peppers, raw	1.00
Boiled prawns	1.10
Green peppers, raw	1.20
Baked beans	1.40
Wholemeal spaghetti, boiled	1.40
White bread	1.60
Spinach, boiled	1.70
Boiled egg	1.90
White self-raising flour	2.00
Brazil nuts	2.50
Peanuts	2.50
Leg of lamb, cooked	2.70
Wholemeal bread	2.70
Topside of beef, cooked	2.80
Almonds	3.00
Soya beans, boiled	3.00

Lentils, boiled	3.50
Hovis	3.70
Wholemeal flour	3.90
Muesli	5.60
Cornflakes	6.70
Rice Krispies	6.70
Soya flour	6.90

MAGNESIUM
Milligrams per 100 g (3.5 oz)

Butter	2.00
Cox's apple	6.00
Turnip, baked	6.00
Young carrots	6.00
Tomato	7.00
Cottage cheese	9.00
Orange	10.00
Full-fat milk	11.00
White rice, boiled	11.00
Semi-skimmed milk	11.00
Skimmed milk	12.00
Boiled egg	12.00
Cornflakes	14.00
Potatoes, boiled	14.00
Red peppers, raw	14.00
White pasta	15.00
Wholemeal spaghetti, boiled	15.00
White self-raising flour	20.00
Green peppers, raw	24.00
Roast chicken	24.00
Topside of beef, cooked	24.00
White bread	24.00
Avocado	25.00
Cheddar cheese	25.00
Grilled cod	26.00
Roast turkey	27.00
Leg of lamb, cooked	28.00
Baked salmon	29.00
Baked beans	31.00
Spinach, boiled	31.00
Grilled herring	32.00
Banana	34.00
Lentils, boiled	34.00
Boiled prawns	42.00
Wholemeal spaghetti, boiled	42.00
Brown rice, boiled	43.00
Hovis	56.00
Soya beans, boiled	63.00

Wholemeal bread	76.00
Muesli	85.00
Wholemeal flour	120.00
Peanuts	210.00
Soya flour	240.00
Almonds	270.00
Brazil nuts	410.00

SELENIUM
Micrograms per 100 g (3.5 oz)

Full-fat milk	1.00
Semi-skimmed milk	1.00
Skimmed milk	1.00
Baked beans	2.00
Cornflakes	2.00
Orange	2.00
Peanuts	3.00
Almonds	4.00
Cottage cheese	4.00
White rice	4.00
White self-raising flour	4.00
Soya beans, boiled	5.00
Boiled egg	11.00
Cheddar cheese	12.00
White bread	28.00
Wholemeal bread	35.00
Lentils, boiled	40.00
Wholemeal flour	53.00

ZINC

Milligrams per 100 g (3.5 oz)

Butter	0.10
Pear	0.10
Orange	0.10
Red peppers, raw	0.10
Banana	0.20
Young carrots	0.20
Cornflakes	0.30
Potatoes, boiled	0.30
Avocado	0.40
Full-fat milk	0.40
Skimmed milk	0.40
Green peppers, raw	0.40
Semi-skimmed milk	0.40
Baked beans	0.50
Grilled cod	0.50
Grilled herring	0.50
White pasta	0.50
Tomatoes	0.50
Cottage cheese	0.60
Spinach, boiled	0.60
White bread	0.60
White self-raising flour	0.60
Brown rice	0.70
White rice	0.70
Soya beans, boiled	0.90
Wholemeal spaghetti, boiled	1.10
Boiled egg	1.30
Lentils, boiled	1.40
Roast chicken	1.50
Boiled prawns	1.60
Wholemeal bread	1.80
Hovis	2.10
Cheddar cheese	2.30
Roast turkey	2.40
Muesli	2.50
Wholemeal flour	2.90
Almonds	3.20
Peanuts	3.50

Brazil nuts	4.20
Leg of lamb, cooked	5.30
Topside of beef, cooked	5.50

ESSENTIAL FATTY ACIDS

Exact amounts of these fats are hard to quantify. Good sources for the two families of essential fatty acids are given.

OMEGA 6 SERIES ESSENTIAL FATTY ACIDS

Sunflower oil
Rape seed oil
Corn oil
Almonds
Walnuts
Brazil nuts
Sunflower seeds
Soya products including Tofu

OMEGA 3 SERIES ESSENTIAL FATTY ACIDS

Mackerel
Herring } fresh cooked or smoked/pickled
Salmon
Walnuts and walnut oil
rape seed oil
Soya products and soy bean oil

Appendix II

References

CHAPTER 1
PLANNING A HEALTHY BABY

Conover, E. A., 'Guarding against foetal toxins', RN, July, 1994.
Barker, D. J. P., *Mothers, Babies, and Disease in Later Life*, British *Medical Journal*, Publishing Group, 1994.

CHAPTER 2
THE EFFECT OF NUTRITION ON BIRTH WEIGHT AND DEVELOPMENT

Barker, D. J. P., *Mothers, Babies, and Disease in Later Life*, British *Medical Journal*, Publishing Group, 1994.
Wynn, M., Wynn, Arthur, 'New thoughts on maternal nutrition', The Caroline Walker Lecture 1993, published by the Caroline Walker Trust.
Lucas, A., 'Programming by Early Nutrition in Man', in Bock, G. R., Whelan, J., eds, *The Childhood Environment and Adult Disease*, John Wiley & Sons, 1991; 38–55.
Widdowson, E. M., McCance, R. A., 'A review: new thoughts on growth', *Pediatric Research*, 1975; 9: 154–6.
Widdowson, E. M., McCance, R. A., 'The effect of finite periods of undernutrition at different ages on the composition and subsequent development of the rat', Proceed-

ings of the Royal Society of London (Biol.), 1963; 158: 329–42.

Barker, D. J. P. *et al*, 'Weight in infancy and death from ischaemic heart disease', *The Lancet*, 1989; ii: 577–80.

Osmond, C., Barker, D. J. P. *et al*, 'Early growth and death from cardiovascular disease in women', *British Medical Journal*, 1993; 307: 1519–24.

Barker, D. J. P. *et al*, 'Foetal nutrition and cardiovascular disease in adult life', *The Lancet*, 1993; 341: 938–41.

Barker, D. J. P. *et al*, 'Growth in utero, blood pressure in childhood and adult life, and mortality from cardiovascular disease', *British Medical Journal*, 1989; 298: 564–7.

Barker, D. J. P. *et al*, 'Foetal and placental size and risk of hypertension in adult life', *British Medical Journal*, 1990; 301: 259–62.

Law, C. M. *et al*, 'Initiation of hypertension in utero and its amplification throughout life', *British Medical Journal*, 1993; 306: 24–7.

Barker, D. J. P. *et al*, 'The relation of fetal length, ponderal index and head circumference to blood pressure and the risk of hypertension in adult life', *Paediatric and Perinatal Epidemiology*, 1992; 6: 35–44.

Barker, D. J. P. *et al*, 'Foetal nutrition and cardiovascular disease in adult life', *The Lancet*, 1993; 341: 938–41.

Godfrey, K. M. *et al*, 'Relation of fingerprints and shape of the palm to foetal growth and adult blood pressure', *British Medical Journal*, 1993; 307: 405–9.

Phipps, K., Barker, D. J. P. *et al*, 'Foetal growth and impaired glucose tolerance in men and women', *Diabetologia*, 1993; 36: 225–8.

McCance, D. R. *et al*, 'Birthweight and non-insulin dependent diabetes: "thrifty geotype", "thrifty phenotype" or "surviving small baby genotype" ', *British Medical Journal*, 1994; 308: 942–5.

Weinkove, C. *et al*, 'Insulin release and pancreatic islet

volume in malnourished rats', *South African Medical Journal*, 1974; 48: 1888.

Snoeck, A. *et al*, 'Effect of a low protein diet during pregnancy on the fetal rat endocrine pancreas', *Biology of the Neonate*, 1990; 5: 107–18.

Hales, C. N., Barker, D. J. P., 'Type 2 (non-insulin dependent) diabetes mellitus: the thrifty phenotype hypothesis', *Diabetologia*, 1992; 35: 595–601.

Strachan, D. P., 'Do chesty children become chesty adults?', *Archives of Diseases of Childhood*, 1990; 65: 161–2.

Downham, M. A. P. S. *et al*, 'Breast feeding protects against respiratory syncytial virus infections', *British Medical Journal*, 1976; ii: 274–6.

Pullan, C. R. *et al*, 'Breast feeding and respiratory syncytial virus infection', *British Medical Journal*, 1980; 281: 1034–8.

Pagtakhan, R. D. *et al*, 'Sex differences in growth patterns of the airways and lung parenchyma in children', *Journal of Applied Physiology*, 1984; 56: 1204–10.

Tepper, R. S. *et al*, 'Physiologic growth and development of the lung during the first year of life', *American Review of Respiratory Disease*, 1986; 134: 513–19.

Gold, D. R. *et al*, 'Acute lower respiratory illness in childhood as a predictor of lung function and chronic respiratory symptoms', *American Review of Respiratory Disease*, 1989; 140: 877–84.

CHAPTER 3
ESSENTIAL NUTRIENTS FOR YOU AND YOUR BABY

Innis, S. M., 'Essential fatty acids in growth and development', *Progress in Lipid Research*, 1991; 30: 39–103.

Clandinin, M. T. *et al*, 'Requirements of newborn infants for long chain polyunsaturated fatty acids', *Acta Paediatrica Scandinavia*, 1989; 351: 63–71.

Koletzbo, B., Schundt, E., Brenner H. R. *et al*, 'Effects of dietary long chain polyunsaturated fatty acids on the essential fatty acid status of premature infants', *European Journal of Pediatrics*, 1989; 148: 669–75.

Koletzbo, B., 'Fats for brains', *European Journal of Clinical Nutrition*, 1992; 46; Suppl. 1: S51–62.

Lucas, A. *et al*, 'Breast milk and subsequent intelligence quotient in children born preterm', *The Lancet*, 1 Feb 1992; 339(8788): 261–4.

Cant, A., Silay, J., Horrobin, D., 'The effect of maternal supplementation with linoleic and gamma-linolenic acids on the fat composition and content of human milk: a placebo-controlled trial', *Journal of Nutritional Science and Vitaminology*, 1991; 37: 573–9.

Makrides, M. *et al*, 'Are long chain polyunsaturated fatty acids essential nutrients in infancy?', *The Lancet*, 1995; 345: 1463–8.

CHAPTER 4
HOW TO IMPROVE YOUR FERTILITY

Healey, D. L., Trounson, A. O., Andersen, A. N., 'Female infertility: causes and treatment', *The Lancet*, 1994; 343: 1539–44.

Editorial, 'Declining fertility: egg or uterus?', *The Lancet*, 1991; 338: 285–6.

Rowe, P. J., Comhaire, F. H., Hargreave, T. B., Mellows, H. J., 'World Health Organisation Manual for the Standard Investigation and Diagnosis of the Infertile Couple', Cambridge University Press, 1993.

Calloway, D. H., 'Nutrition and reproductive function and men', nutrition abstracts and reviews in *Clinical Nutrition*, Series A, 1983; 53(5): 361–80.

Skakkebaek, N. E., Giwercman, A., de Krester, D., 'Pathogenesis and management of male infertility', *The Lancet*, 1994; 343: 1473–9.

Hargreave, T. B., 'Non-specific treatment to improve fertility', in *Male Fertility*, ed. Hargreave, T. B., Springer-Verlag, 1983, pp. 227–45.

CHAPTER 5
THE TRUTH ABOUT SOCIAL POISONS

Spohr, H. L. *et al*, 'Prenatal alcohol exposure and long-term developmental consequences', *The Lancet*, 1993; 341: 907–10.

Macdonald, A. D. *et al*, 'Cigarette, alcohol and coffee consumption and spontaneous abortion', *American Journal of Public Health*, 1992; 82: 85–7.

Aldridge, A. *et al*, 'The disposition of caffeine during and after pregnancy', seminars in *Perinatology*, 1981; 5: 310–14.

Brooke, O. G. *et al*, 'Effects on birth weight of smoking, alcohol, caffeine, socio-economic factors and psychosocial stress', *British Medical Journal*, 1989; 298: 795–801.

Fogelman, K. R., Manor, O., 'Smoking in pregnancy and development in early childhood', *British Medical Journal*, 1988; 297: 1233–6.

Haste, F. M. *et al*, 'The effect of nutritional intake on outcome of pregnancy in smokers and non-smokers', *British Journal of Nutrition*, 1991; 65: 347–54.

Beaulac-Baillargeon, L., Desrosiers, C., 'Caffeine and cigarette interaction on fetal growth', *American Journal of Obstetrics and Gynaecology*, 1987; 157: 1236–40.

Nieburg, P. *et al*, 'The fetal tobacco syndrome', *Journal of the American Medical Association*, 1985; 253: 2998–9.

Stirling, H. F. *et al*, 'Passive smoking in utero: its effects on neonatal appearance', *British Medical Journal*, 1987; 295: 627–8.

Brewley, B. R., 'Smoking in pregnancy', *British Medical Journal*, 1984; 288: 424–6.

Dolan-Mullen, P. *et al*, 'A meta-analysis of randomized trials of prenatal smoking cessation interventions', *American Journal of Obstetrics and Gynaecology*, 1994; 1328–34.

Czeizel, A. E. *et al*, 'Smoking during pregnancy and congenital limb deficiency', *British Medical Journal*, 1994; 308: 1473–6.

Editorial, 'Maternal smoking affects blood pressure in offspring', *Archives of Diseases in Childhood*, 1995; 72: 120–4.

Infante-Rivard, C. *et al*, 'Fetal loss associated with caffeine intake before and during pregnancy', *Journal of the American Medical Association*, 1993; 270: 2940–3.

Wei, Dr M., 'Foetal loss and caffeine intake', letter to editor, *Journal of the American Medical Association*, 6 July 1994; 272, No. 1.

Ashton, C. H., 'Caffeine and health', *British Medical Journal*, 21 November 1987; 295: 6609: 1294.

Griffiths, R. R. *et al*, 'Human coffee drinking: manipulation of concentration and caffeine dose', *Journal of Experimental and Analytical Behaviour*, 1986; 45: 133–48.

Eriksson, M., Zetterstrom, R., 'Amphetamine addiction during pregnancy: 10-year follow-up', *Acta Paediatrica Scandinavia*, 1994; Suppl. 404: 27–31.

Smit, B. J. *et al*, 'Cocaine use in pregnancy in Amsterdam', *Acta Paediatrica Scandinavia*, 1994; Suppl. 404: 32–5.

van Baar, A. L. *et al*, 'Development after prenatal exposure to cocaine, heroin and methadone', *Acta Paediatrica Scandinavia*, 1994; Suppl. 404: 40–6.

Soepatmi, S., 'Developmental outcomes of children of mothers dependent on heroin or heroin/methadone during pregnancy', *Acta Paediatrica Scandinavia*, 1994; Suppl. 404: 36–9.

Stenchever, M. A, *et al*, 'Chromosome breakages in uses of marijuana', *American Journal of Obstetrics and Gynaecology*, 1974; 118: 106–13.

CHAPTER 6
FACTFILE ON MISCARRIAGE

Regan, L., 'Recurrent miscarriage', *British Medical Journal*, 1991; 302: 543–4.

Tulppala, N. *et al*, 'Thromboxane dominance and prosta-cyclin deficiency in habitual abortion', *The Lancet*, 1991; 337: 879–81.

Hay, T. E., Lamont, R. P., Taylor-Robinson, D. *et al*, 'Abnormal bacterial colonization of the genital tract and subsequent pre-term delivery and late miscarriage', *British Medical Journal*, 1994; 308: 295–8.

CHAPTER 8
PREGNANCY: YOUR QUESTIONS ANSWERED

Barker, D. J. P., *Mothers, Babies and Disease in Later Life*, British Medical Journal, Publishing, 1994.

Sandstead, H. H. *et al*, 'Human zinc deficiency, endocrine manifestations and response to treatment', *The American Journal of Clinical Nutrition*, Vol. 20, No. 5, May 1967; 4232–442.

Snowise, N., 'Dietary advice in pregnancy', *Update*, 15 May 1994; 804–6.

While you are pregnant: safe eating and how to avoid infection from food and animals, Department of Health and the Central Office of Information, HMSO, 1991.

The diagnosis and treatment of suspected listeriosis in pregnancy, Standing Medical Advisory Group, HMSO, 1992.

Vitamin A and pregnancy, Chief Medical Officer, Department of Health letters to all doctors, October 1990 and November 1993.

Maternal and Foetal Nutrition, National Dairy Council, Fact File number 11, 1994.

Maternal weight gain and its usefulness, Clinical Reviews, 12 April 1991; 27–8.

Daws, M. G. *et al*, 'Patterns of maternal weight gain in pregnancy', *British Journal of Obstetrics and Gynaecology*, 1991; 98: 195–201.

Dawes, M. G. *et al*, 'Repeated measurement of maternal weight during pregnancy. Is it a useful practice?' *British Journal of Obstetrics and Gynaecology*, 1991; 98: 189–94.

'Routine Iron Supplements in Pregnancy are Unnecessary', *British National Formulary*, April 1994.

Barker, D. J. P. *et al*, 'Fetal and placental size and the risk of hypertension in adult life', *British Medical Journal*, 1990; 301: 259–62.

Godfrey, K. M., Redman, C. W. G., Barker, D. J. P., Osmond, C., 'The effect of maternal anaemia and iron deficiency on the ratio of foetal weight to placental weight', *British Journal of Obstetrics and Gynaecology*, 1991; 98: 886–91.

'Anaemia, iron and placental weight', Clinical Reviews, November 1991; 23–4.

Hemminki, E., Rimpela, U., 'A randomized comparison of routine versus selective iron supplementation during pregnancy', *Journal of the American College of Nutrition*, 1991; 10: 1: 3–10.

Hemminki, E., Rimpela, U., 'Iron supplementation, maternal packed cell volume, and fetal growth', *Archives of Disease in Childhood*, 1991; 66: 423–5.

Clark, N., Fisk, M., 'Minimal compliance with the Department of Health recommendation for routine folate prophylaxis to prevent fetal neural tube defects', *British Journal of Obstetrics and Gynaecology*, August 1994; 101: 709–10.

Czeizel, A. E., Dudas, I., 'Prevention of the first occurrence of neural tube defects by periconceptual vitamin supplementation', *New England Journal of Medicine*, 1992; 327: 1832–5.

Czeizel, A. E., 'Periconceptional multivitamin supplementation in prevention of congenital abnormalities', *Maternal and Child Health*, December 1994; 381–4.

UK Department of Health, Health Publicity Unit, 'Folic acid and prevention of neural tube defects', *The Lancet*, 1993; 341: 46.

Department of Health, *Folic Acid and the Prevention of Neural Tube Defects: Reports from an Expert Advisory Group*, HMSO, 1992.

'Folic Acid to Prevent Neural Tube Defects', *British National Formulary*, April 1994.

Rosenberg, I. H., 'Folic acid and neural-tube defects – time for action?', *New England Journal of Medicine*, 1992; 372: 26: 1875–7.

Wald, N. *et al*, MRC Vitamin Study Research Group, 'Prevention of neural tube defects', *The Lancet*, 1991; 338: 131–7.

Kirke, P. N., Molloy, A. M., Daly, L. E. *et al*, 'Maternal plasma folate and vitamin B12 are independent risk factors for neural tube defects', *Quarterly Journal of Medicine*, 1993; 86: 703–8.

Belluomini, J. *et al*, 'Acupressure for nausea and vomiting of pregnancy: a randomized, blinded study', *Journal of Obstetrics and Gynaecology*, 1994; 84: 245–8.

Laroque, B. *et al*, 'Effects on birth weight of alcohol and caffeine consumption during pregnancy', *American Journal of Epidemiology*, 1993; 137; (9): 941–50.

Spohr H.L., *et al*, 'Prenatal alcohol exposure and long-term developmental consequences', *The Lancet*, 1993; 341: 907–10.

Brewley, B.R., 'Smoking in pregnancy', *British Medical Journal*, February 1984; 288: 424–6.

Dolan-Mullen, P. *et al*, 'A meta-analysis of randomized trials of prenatal smoking cessation interventions', *American Journal of Obstetrics and Gynaecology*, 1994; 1328–34.

Czeizel, A. E. *et al*, 'Smoking during pregnancy and congenital limb deficiency', *British Medical Journal*, 1994; 308: 1473–6.

Editorial, 'Maternal smoking affects blood pressure in offspring', *Archives of Diseases in Childhood*, 1995; 72: 120–4.

Infante-Rivard, C. *et al*, 'Fetal loss associated with caffeine intake before and during pregnancy', *Journal of the American Medical Association*, 1993; 270: 2940–3.

Wei, Dr M., 'Foetal loss and caffeine intake', letter to editor, *Journal of the American Medical Association*, 6 July 1994; 272, No. 1.

Claoo, J. F., 'The effects of maternal exercise on early pregnancy outcome', *American Journal of Obstetrics and Gynaecology*, 1989; 161: 1453–7.

Kitzinger, S., *The National Childbirth Trust Book of Pregnancy, Birth and Parenthood*, Oxford University Press, 1993.

CHAPTER 10
DIET FOR PREGNANCY

Dietary Reference Values of Food Energy and Nutrients for the United Kingdom, Department of Health Report of the Panel on Dietary Reference Values of the Committee on Medical Aspects of Food Policy, HMSO, 1991.

McCance and Widdowson, *The Composition of Foods*, HMSO, 1976, supplements 1985, 1988, 1989, 1990, 1991 and 1992.

CHAPTER 12
THE VALUE OF EXERCISE

Claoo, J. F., 'The effects of maternal exercise on early pregnancy outcome', *American Journal of Obstetrics and Gynaecology*, 1989; 161: 1453–7.

CHAPTER 13
THE BENEFITS OF RELAXATION

Sutcliffe, J., *The Complete Book of Relaxation Techniques*, Headline, 1992.
Maxwell-Hudson, C., *The Complete Book of Massage*, Dorling Kindersley, 1990.

CHAPTERS 17, 18, 19
WEANING, STAGES ONE TO THREE

'Weaning and the Weaning Diet', Department of Health Report of the Working Group on the Weaning Diet of the Committee on Medical Aspects of Food Policy, HMSO, 1994.

Appendix III

Recommended Reading List

Note: UK, USA and A denote the following books are available in Great Britain, the United States of America and Australia.

GENERAL HEALTH
1. *The Vitality Diet*
   by Dr Alan and Maryon Stewart
   (published by Thorsons) UK A
2. *Coming off Tranquillizers*
   by Dr Shirley Trickett
   (published by Thorsons) UK USA A (Lothian Publishing Co.)
3. *The Migraine Revolution – The Drug-Free Solution*
   by Dr John Mansfield
   (published by Thorsons) UK USA A (Lothian Publishing Co.)
4. *Nutritional Medicine*
   by Dr Stephen Davies and Dr Alan Stewart
   (published by Pan Books) UK A
5 *Pain-free Periods*
   by Stella Weller
   (published by Thorsons) UK
6. *Osteoporosis*

by Kathleen Mayes
(published by Thorsons) UK
7. *Beat PMS Through Diet*
by Maryon Stewart
(published by Vermilion) UK
8. *Beat IBS Through Diet*
by Maryon Stewart and Dr Alan Stewart
(published by Vermilion) UK
9. *Tired All the Time*
by Dr Alan Stewart
(published by Optima) UK A
10. *Natural Hormone Health*
by Arabella Melville
(published by Thorsons) UK USA A

DIET
1. *The New Raw Energy*
by Leslie and Susannah Kenton
(published by Vermilion) UK A (Doubleday)
2. *Foresight Index Number Decoder (Packet Food Additive Dictionary)*
price £1.35 + 20p p&p, available from Foresight (address in Useful Addresses List) UK
3. *The Reluctant Vegetarian Cook*
by Simon Hope
(published by William Heinemann) UK
4. *The Single Vegan*
by Leah Leneman
(published by Thorsons) UK
5. *Organic Consumer Guide/Food you can trust*
Edited by David Mabey and Alan and Jackie Gear
(published by Thorsons) UK USA A
6. *Beat Sugar Craving*
by Maryon Stewart
(published by Vermilion) UK

7. *Whole Earth Cookbook*
   by Hilary Meth
   (published by Vermilion) UK

DRUGS
1. *What Do You Know About Drugs?*
   by Sanders & Myers
   (published by Gloucester Press, £8.99)
2. *Forbidden Drugs – Understanding Drugs and How People Take Them* by Robson
   (published by Oxford University Press, £9.99)

SMOKING
1. *Easy Way to Stop Smoking*
   by Allen Carr
   (published by Penguin, £6.99)

STRESS
1. *Self Help for Your Nerves*
   by Dr Claire Weekes
   (published by HarperCollins) UK USA
2. *Stress Wise*
   by Dr Terry Looker and Dr Olga Gregson
   (published by Headway) UK

PREGNANCY AND BABY BOOKS
1. *The Book of Yoga*
   by The Sivananda Yoga Centre
   (published by Ebury) UK USA
2. *The Complete Book of Relaxation Techniques*
   by Jenny Sutcliffe
   (published by Headline) UK
3. *The Complete Book of Massage*
   by Clare Maxwell-Hudson
   (published by Dorling Kindersley) UK

4. *A Child is Born*
   by Lennart Nilsson
   (published by Doubleday) UK USA A
5. *Planning for a Healthy Baby*
   by Belinda Barnes and Suzanne Gail Bradley (Foresight)
   (published by Vermilion) UK
6. *Green Babies*
   by Penny Stanway
   (published by Century) UK USA
7. *The National Childbirth Trust Book of Pregnancy, Birth and Parenthood*
   by Sheila Kitzinger
   (published by Oxford University Press) UK USA
8. *The National Childbirth Trust Book of Breast-feeding*
   by Mary Smale
   (published by Vermilion) UK USA
9. *Your Choices for Pregnancy and Childbirth*
   by Helen Lewison
   (published by Ebury) UK USA
10. *Breast is Best*
    by Doctors Penny and Andrew Stanway
    (published by Pan Books)

YOGA
1. *Preparing for Birth With Yoga*
   by Janet Balakas
   (published by Element, £14.99)
2. *Instant Stress Cure*
   by Lyn Marshall
   (published by Vermilion, £8.99)

APPENDIX IV

Further Help and Telephone Advice Lines

If you would like to attend the Women's Nutritional Advisory Service (WNAS) Clinic, or need further details about our telephone and postal courses of treatment, you can write to the WNAS at the address below with a large self-addressed envelope and four separate, loose, first-class stamps. Please state clearly that you wish further information on pregnancy and breast-feeding, as we help women with all sorts of other problems.

I should also be interested to hear about your success using the recommendations in this book.

The address to write to is:

Women's Nutritional Advisory Service
PO Box 268
Lewes
East Sussex BN7 2QN

All clinic appointments are booked on 01273 487366.
We also have a number of advice lines which you may be interested in listening to:

Get Fit for Pregnancy and Breast-feeding   0839 556608
Overcome PMS Naturally   0839 556600

The PMS Diet Line	0839 556601
Overcome Menopause Naturally	0839 556602
The Menopause Diet Line	0839 556603
Beat Sugar Craving	0839 556604
The Vitality Diet Line	0839 556605
Overcoming Breast Tenderness	0839 556606
Overcome Period Pains Naturally	0839 556607
Skin, Nail and Hair Signs of Deficiency	0839 556609
Improve Libido Naturally	0839 556610
Beat Irritable Bowel Syndrome	0839 556611
Overcome Fatigue	0839 556612
Beat Migraine Naturally	0839 556613
Overcome Ovulation Pain	0839 556614
Directory	0839 556615

Appendix V

Useful Addresses

GENERAL HEALTH

ASH (Action on Smoking and Health)
109 Gloucester Place
London W1H 4EJ
Tel: 0171 935 3519

Alcoholics Anonymous (AA)
General Services Office
PO Box 1
Stonebow House
Stonebow
York YO1 2NJ
Tel: 01904 644026

Alcohol Counselling Prevention Services
34 Electric Lane
London SW9 8JT
Tel: 0171 737 3579

Anorexia and Bulimia Nervosa Association
24 Westmoreland Road
Barnes
London SW13 9RY

Tel: 0181 748 3994

Association for Spina Bifida and Hydrocephalus
ASBAH House
42 Park Road
Peterborough
Cambridgeshire PE1 2UQ
Tel: 01733 555988

College of Health
St Margaret's House
21 Old Ford Road
London E2 9PL
Tel: 0181 983 1225

Down's Syndrome Association
155 Mitcham Road
London SW17 9PG
Tel: 0181 682 4001

Drugaid
1 Neville Street
Cardiff CF1 8LP
Tel: 01222 383313

Eating Disorders Association
Sackville Place
44 Magdalen Street
Norwich
Norfolk NR3 1JU
Tel: *Helpline* 01603 621414
         Youth 01603 765050
         Recorded message 0891 615466

Foresight
Association for the Promotion of Preconceptual Care
28 The Paddock
Godalming
Surrey GU7 1XD
Tel: 01483 427839

Allergy Care
Pollards Yard
Wood Street
Taunton
Somerset TA1 1UP
Tel: 01823 325023

Friends of the Earth Ltd
26–28 Underwood Street
London N1 7JQ
Tel: 0171 490 1555

Herpes Association
41 North Road
London N7 9DP
Tel: 0171 609 9061

Migraine Trust
45 Great Ormond Street
London WC1N 3HZ
Tel: 0171 278 2676

National AIDS Helpline
Tel: 0800 567 123

Pelvic Inflammatory Disease Network
Women's Health
52 Featherstone Street

London EC1Y 8RT
Tel: 0171 251 6580

QUIT
Victory House
170 Tottenham Court Road
London W1P 0HA
Smokers' Quitline: 0171 487 3000 (09.30–17.30 daily)

Samaritans
General Office of the Samaritans
10 The Grove
Slough
Berkshire SL1 1QP
Tel: 01753 532713

The Soil Association
86 Colston Street
Bristol BS1 5BB
Tel: 0117 9290661

The Shiatsu Therapy Centre
No permanent address yet but telephone:
Tel: 01505 682889

Support after Termination of Pregnancy for Abnormality
73–75 Charlotte Street
London W1P 1LB
Tel: 0171 631 0280
Helpline: 0171 631 0285

Toxoplasmosis Trust
Room 26
61–71 Collier Street
London N1 9BE

Helpline: 0171 713 0599

The Vegetarian Society
Parkdale
Dunham Road
Altrincham
Cheshire WA14 4QG
Tel: 0161 928 0793

Vegan Society
Donald Watson House
7 Battle Road
St Leonards-on-Sea
East Sussex TN3Y 7AA
Tel: 01424 427393

WOMEN'S HEALTH

Association for Improvements in Maternity Services (AIMS)
40 Kingswood Avenue
London NW6 6LS

Association for Post-Natal Illness
25 Jerdan Place
Fulham
London SW6 1BE
Tel: 0171 386 0868

British Pregnancy Advisory Service
Austy Manor
Wootton Wawen
Solihull
West Midlands B95 6BX
Tel: 01564 793225

Brook Advisory Centre
Central Offices
153a East Street
London SE17 2SD
Tel: 0171 763 9660

Centre for Pregnancy Nutrition
The University of Sheffield
Department of Obstetrics and Gynaecology
Clinical Sciences Centre
Northern General Hospital
Herries Road
Sheffield S5 7AU
Tel: 0114 243 4343 ext 4888

The National Endometriosis Society
Suite 50
Westminster Palace Gardens
1–7 Artillery Road
London SW1P 1RR
Tel: 0171 222 2776

Family Planning Information Service
27–35 Mortimer Street
London W1N 7RJ
Tel: 0171 636 7866

International Planned Parenthood Federation
Regent's College
Inner Circle
Regent's Park
London NW1 4NS
Tel: 0171 486 0741

LIFE
Life House
Newbold Terrace
Leamington Spa
Warwickshire CV32 4EA
Tel: 01926 311511

Maternity Alliance
15 Britannia Street
London WC1X 9JN
Tel: 0171 837 1265

Miscarriage Association
c/o Clayton Hospital
Northgate
Wakefield
West Yorkshire WF1 3JS
Tel: 01924 200799

National Association for Maternal and Child Care Welfare
1 South Audley Street
London W1Y 6JS

National Childbirth Trust
Alexandra House
Oldham Terrace
London W3 6NH
Tel: 0181 992 8637

The National Osteoporosis Society
PO Box 10
Radstock
Bath BA3 3YB
Tel: 01761 471771

Natural Family Planning Centre
Birmingham Maternity Hospital
Queen Elizabeth Medical Centre
Edgbaston
Birmingham B15 2TG
Tel: 0121 627 2698

Natural Family Planning Service
Catholic Marriage Advisory Council
Clitherow House
1 Blythe Mews
Blythe Road
London W14 0NW
Tel: 0171 371 1341

Pregnancy Advisory Service
11–13 Charlotte Street
London W1P 1HD
Tel: 0171 637 8962

WellBeing
27 Sussex Place
Regent's Park
London NW1 4SP
Tel: 0171 723 9296

Womanschoice
4 Butler's Grove
Basildon
Essex SS16 6HW
Tel: 01268 543069

Women's Health and Reproductive Rights Information Centre
52 Featherstone Street
London EC1Y 8RT

Tel: 0171 251 6580

The Women's Nutritional Advisory Service
PO Box 268
Lewes
East Sussex BN7 2QN
Tel: 01273 487366

ALTERNATIVE HEALTH

British Homeopathic Association
27a Devonshire Street
London W1N 1RJ
Tel: 0171 935 2163

British Acupuncture Association
34 Alderney Street
London SW1V 4EU
Tel: 0171 834 1012

British School of Osteopathy
Administration and Clinics
1–4 Suffolk Street
London SW1Y 4HG
Tel: 0171 930 9254

Institute for Complementary Medicine
PO Box 194
London SE16 1QZ
Tel: 0171 237 5165

The European School of Osteopathy
104 Tonbridge Road
Maidstone
Kent ME16 8SL

Tel: 01622 671558

AUSTRALIA – ACT

Abortion and Counselling Service
Tel: 06 247 8070

Family Planning Association ACT
Childers Street
Canberra City
ACT 2601
Tel: 06 247 3077

Family Planning Australia
PO Box 9026
Deakin
ACT 2600
or
Lua Building
Suite 3, First Floor
39 Geils Court
Deakin
ACT 2600
Tel: 06 285 1244
Fax: 06 282 5298

Natural Family Planning
PO Box 3167
Manuka
ACT 2601
Tel: 06 239 7700

Pregnancy Advisory Service
Childers Street
Canberra City

ACT 2601
Tel: 06 248 6222

Pregnancy Support Service ACT Inc
PO Box 476
Civic Square
ACT 2608
Tel: 06 248 5050

SANDS (Stillbirth and Neonatal Death Support)
PO Box 204
Curtin
ACT 2605

AIDS Action Council
Tel: 06 257 2855

QUITS
Tel: 06 282 3452

ACT Women's Health Service
Tel: 06 205 1078

Alcohol and Drug Service
Tel: 06 205 1323

Canberra Women's Health Centre
Tel: 06 290 2166

Childbirth Education Association
Tel: 06 257 4909

AUSTRALIAN STATES

New South Wales
Leichhardt Women's Health Centre
Tel: 02 560 3011

Northern Territory
Darwin Women's Information Centre
Tel: 089 277 166

Queensland
Brisbane Women's Health Centre
Tel: 07 839 9988

South Australia
Adelaide Women's Health Centre
Tel: 08 267 5366

Tasmania
Hobart Women's Health Centre
Tel: 002 313 212

Victoria
Healthsharing Women
Tel: 03 663 3544

Western Australia
Whitford Women's Health Centre
Tel: 09 344 8012

CANADA

Planned Parenthood Federation Canada
1 Nicholas Street
Suite 430

Ottawa
Ontario
K1N 7B7
Tel: 001 613 2384474
Fax: 001 613 2381162

NEW ZEALAND

New Zealand Family Planning Association Inc
2nd Floor, Castrol House
CNR Dixon
Victoria Street
Wellington
Tel: 00 644 3844349
Fax: 00 644 3828356

SOUTH AFRICA

Association for Dietetics
PO Box 4309
Randburg
2125
South Africa

Appendix VI

Nutritional Supplement Suppliers

UK
Efamol Ltd
Wharf House
Wharf Road
Guildford
Surrey GU1 4RP
Tel: 01483 304441
    01483 304437
Supplies: Efamol

Larkhall Natural Health/Greenfarm
225–229 Putney Bridge Road
London SW1Y 2PY
Tel: 0181 871 0401
Supplies: A wide range of vitamins, minerals and specialised food including Trufree flour

Nature's Best Health Products Ltd
1 Lamberts Road
Tunbridge Wells
Kent TN2 3EQ
Tel: 01892 534143
Supplies: A wide range of vitamins and minerals. Also Optivite

Nature's Own
203–205 West Malvern Road
West Malvern
Worcs WR14 4BB
Tel: 01684 892555
Supplies: A wide range of vitamins and minerals

Boots the Chemist
All branches
Supplies: Cream of magnesia, Efamol and Efamol Marine

Practitioners can buy Chromium GTF from Lamberts.

AUSTRALIA
The NNFA have lists of all supplement stockists and retailers in Australia, if you have any difficulties in obtaining supplements. PMT Formula is available from Blackmores, 23 Roseberry Street, Balgowlah, NSW 2093, Australia (*Tel*: 02 951 0111).

NEW ZEALAND
Again the NNFA have lists of all supplement stockists and retailers in New Zealand, if you have any difficulties in obtaining supplements. PMT Formula is available from Blackmores, 2 Parkhead Place, North Harbour, Albany, Auckland, New Zealand (*Tel*: 09 415 8585).

INDEX

302